THE EVERYTHING® PALEO PREGNANCY BOOK

Dear Reader,

Since discovering a Paleo way of eating, I have done everything in my power to shout my "real food message" from the mountaintops. There is so much confusing (and often conflicting) diet information out there, and it was a revelation to learn that it is possible to be healthy and thrive by eating the way our ancestors did. Even before pregnancy, I felt stronger, more energetic, and more in tune with my body than I ever had before. Once I learned that I was pregnant, following a Paleo diet became even more important to me because I wanted to nourish my growing baby with nutritious, whole foods.

　　Whether you are new to the Paleo diet or want to learn more about this way of eating to support a happy pregnancy and the healthy growth and development of your baby, The Everything® Paleo Pregnancy Book will give you the knowledge, tools, and confidence to follow a Paleo diet while navigating the ups and downs of pregnancy. Not only will you discover how to manage common symptoms such as fatigue and nausea; you will also learn how to adjust to your new role as "mom," and you'll be treated to dozens of healthy recipes that will provide the nutrients you and your baby need . . . and even a few sweets to satisfy those pregnancy cravings.

　　Wishing you a happy and healthy nine months,

Tarah Chieffi

Welcome to the EVERYTHING® Series!

These handy, accessible books give you all you need to tackle a difficult project, gain a new hobby, comprehend a fascinating topic, prepare for an exam, or even brush up on something you learned back in school but have since forgotten.

You can choose to read an Everything® book from cover to cover or just pick out the information you want from our four useful boxes: e-questions, e-facts, e-alerts, and e-ssentials.

We give you everything you need to know on the subject, but throw in a lot of fun stuff along the way, too.

We now have more than 400 Everything® books in print, spanning such wide-ranging categories as weddings, pregnancy, cooking, music instruction, foreign language, crafts, pets, New Age, and so much more. When you're done reading them all, you can finally say you know Everything®!

QUESTION

Answers to
common questions

FACT

Important snippets
of information

ALERT

Urgent
warnings

ESSENTIAL

Quick
handy tips

PUBLISHER Karen Cooper

MANAGING EDITOR, EVERYTHING® SERIES Lisa Laing

COPY CHIEF Casey Ebert

ASSISTANT PRODUCTION EDITOR Alex Guarco

ACQUISITIONS EDITOR Hillary Thompson

DEVELOPMENT EDITOR Brett Palana-Shanahan

EVERYTHING® SERIES COVER DESIGNER Erin Alexander

Visit the entire Everything® series at *www.everything.com*

THE EVERYTHING®

PALEO PREGNANCY BOOK

The all-natural, nutritious plan
for a healthy pregnancy

Tarah Chieffi

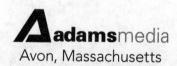

Avon, Massachusetts

This book is dedicated to my loving and supportive husband, Kevin,
who has always believed in me and encouraged me to pursue my dreams.

An Everything® Series Book.
Everything® and everything.com® are registered trademarks of F+W Media, Inc.

Published by Adams Media,
a division of F+W Media, Inc.
57 Littlefield Street, Avon, MA 02322. U.S.A.
www.adamsmedia.com

Contains material adapted and abridged from *The Everything® Pregnancy Nutrition Book* by Kimberly A. Tessmer, copyright © 2005 by F+W Media, Inc., ISBN 10: 1-59337-151-9, ISBN 13: 978-1-59337-151-7; *The Everything® Paleolithic Diet Book* by Jodie Cohen and Gilaad Cohen, copyright © 2011 by F+W Media, Inc., ISBN 10: 1-4405-1206-X, ISBN 13: 978-1-4405-1206-3; *The Everything® Eating Clean Cookbook* by Britt Brandon, copyright © 2012 by F+W Media, Inc., ISBN 10: 1-4405-2999-X, ISBN 13: 978-1-4405-2999-3; *The Everything® Pregnancy Book, 4th Edition* by Paula Ford-Martin, copyright © 2012, 2007, 2003, 1999 by F+W Media, Inc., ISBN 10: 1-4405-2851-9, ISBN 13: 978-1-4405-2851-4; *The Everything® Paleolithic Diet Slow Cooker Cookbook* by Emily Dionne, copyright © 2013 by F+W Media, Inc., ISBN 10: 1-4405-5536-2, ISBN 13: 978-1-4405-5536-7; *The Everything® Guide to Pregnancy Nutrition & Health* by Britt Brandon, copyright © 2013 by F+W Media, Inc., ISBN 10: 1-4405-6011-0, ISBN 13: 978-1-4405-6011-8; *The Everything® Giant Book of Juicing* by Teresa Kennedy, copyright © 2013 by F+W Media, Inc., ISBN 10: 1-4405-5785-3, ISBN 13: 978-1-4405-5785-9; *The Everything® Healthy Green Drinks Book* by Britt Brandon, copyright © 2014 by F+W Media, Inc., ISBN 10: 1-4405-7694-7, ISBN 13: 978-1-4405-7694-2.

ISBN 10: 1-4405-8429-X
ISBN 13: 978-1-4405-8429-9
eISBN 10: 1-4405-8430-3
eISBN 13: 978-1-4405-8430-5

Printed in the United States of America.

10 9 8 7 6 5 4 3 2 1

Library of Congress Cataloging-in-Publication Data
Chieffi, Tarah.
The everything paleo pregnancy book / Tarah Chieffi.
    pages cm
Includes index.
ISBN 978-1-4405-8429-9 (pb) -- ISBN 1-4405-8429-X (pb) -- ISBN 978-1-4405-8430-5 (ebook) -- ISBN 1-4405-8430-3 (ebook)
1. Pregnancy--Nutritional aspects. 2. Prehistoric people--Nutrition. I. Title.
RG559.C45 2015
641.5'6319--dc23
                                        2014033046

Many of the designations used by manufacturers and sellers to distinguish their products are claimed as trademarks. Where those designations appear in this book and F+W Media, Inc. was aware of a trademark claim, the designations have been printed with initial capital letters.

This book is intended as general information only, and should not be used to diagnose or treat any health condition. In light of the complex, individual, and specific nature of health problems, this book is not intended to replace professional medical advice. The ideas, procedures, and suggestions in this book are intended to supplement, not replace, the advice of a trained medical professional. Consult your physician before adopting any of the suggestions in this book, as well as about any condition that may require diagnosis or medical attention. The author and publisher disclaim any liability arising directly or indirectly from the use of this book.

Always follow safety and commonsense cooking protocol while using kitchen utensils, operating ovens and stoves, and handling uncooked food. If children are assisting in the preparation of any recipe, they should always be supervised by an adult.

Cover images © Cedric Carter/skyfotostock/123RF.
Nutritional statistics by Nicole Cormier, RD, LDN.

This book is available at quantity discounts for bulk purchases.
For information, please call 1-800-289-0963.

Contents

Acknowledgments

First and foremost, I am forever grateful to my husband, Kevin, for introducing me to Paleo, encouraging me to share my recipes and experiences with the world, and always being my guinea pig in the kitchen. Thank you to my beautiful son, Avery, for teaching me about unconditional love, always brightening my day, and inspiring me to stay healthy so we can enjoy our adventures together for many, many years to come.

I feel I should also acknowledge a few of the leaders of the Paleo movement: Loren Cordain, Robb Wolf, and Sarah Fragoso. Though there are countless others who have helped to guide me along the way, these are the faces behind the books and websites I turned to most often when I was first introduced to Paleo. I learned from them what it means to live a Paleo lifestyle and how to apply it to my own life.

Finally, thank you to my family and friends for supporting me in all of my endeavors.

Introduction

CONGRATULATIONS, MAMA, YOU'RE PREGNANT! Before you know it, you'll be holding that tiny bundle of joy in your arms. Until then, you are going to get a lot of advice on how to manage your pregnancy—what to buy, what to wear, when to sleep, how to exercise, and even how to eat. If you follow a Paleo diet and know the benefits of following an ancestral way of eating, you may be used to brushing off well-meaning advice when it comes to nutrition. You are already well aware that eating a diet of whole foods such as meat, seafood, vegetables, fruits, and healthy fats can prevent and even reverse disease, improve sleep and energy, and promote optimal body composition. But now that you are pregnant, what you eat and how you care for your body are more important than ever. Your baby needs specific nutrients for proper growth and development, and your nutritional needs are changing, as well. Pregnant women have varying carbohydrate, protein, and fat requirements and also need higher levels of certain vitamins and minerals to support their changing bodies.

You want what is best for your baby, and it is totally normal to have questions and concerns about how much and what you should be eating. This book will give you the scientific evidence that shows how a Paleo diet can help you to meet all of your nutritional needs during pregnancy. It will also provide you with practical tips on getting through each stage of pregnancy and beyond. You will learn which nutrients are most important during pregnancy and where to get them, how to handle common (and not-so-common) pregnancy symptoms and complications, and how to modify your exercise routine. You will also find helpful tips for the postpartum period, such as recovery after delivery, connecting with other new moms, postpartum fitness, bonding with baby, and how to continue with your Paleo lifestyle while tending to the demanding schedule of a newborn. The recipes included in this book are simple, delicious, and often substantial enough that you'll have leftovers for the next day so you can spend a little extra time cuddling your sweet baby. You'll find everything from well-rounded breakfasts to Paleo versions of some of your favorite comfort foods—and healthy snacks and treats to tame your sweet tooth.

The Paleo diet is not about restriction or deprivation. It is about health, longevity, and nourishment. It really isn't even a diet; it is a way of taking control of your health and your life. It is about removing refined, nutrient-depleting foods that can cause digestive distress and promote disease and replacing them with real foods that are minimally processed—foods that make you feel good inside and out. If this way of eating appeals to you, rest assured that you will be providing your baby with everything she needs to thrive by following the advice in this book and that of your health care provider.

So whether you have been following a Paleo diet for years or are totally new to Paleo, this book will become your go-to resource for all things pregnancy and will teach you the benefits to both you and your baby of living a Paleo lifestyle.

CHAPTER 1

Paleo Nutrition and Your Pregnancy

Pregnancy is a time of wonder and amazement as you develop a lifelong bond with your growing baby. It is also your first opportunity to nurture and care for your baby by following a healthy diet, staying active, and allowing yourself time for rest and relaxation. Although you may be going against the grain (so to speak) by following a Paleo lifestyle during pregnancy, you can be sure that this way of eating provides all of the nutrients that you and your baby need as you embark on this journey to motherhood.

An Introduction to the Paleo Lifestyle

If you are new to Paleo, you may be wondering what exactly this lifestyle is all about. According to Dr. Loren Cordain, one of the world's leading experts on the Paleolithic way of eating, "The Paleo Diet is based upon everyday, modern foods that mimic the food groups of our pre-agricultural, hunter-gatherer ancestors." This is the way people ate millions of years ago, before modern farming techniques, food processing plants, and twenty-four-hour drive-throughs.

A lot has changed since then, but not all of it is for the better. Paleolithic man did not suffer from what we now refer to as "diseases of civilization" such as obesity, diabetes, cardiovascular disease, many cancers, autoimmune conditions, and many of the physical and neurological declines associated with aging. Not only that; the number of people today who suffer from digestive issues such as heartburn, ulcers, food sensitivities, Crohn's disease, and celiac disease is on the rise with no end in sight. By removing the highly processed, artificial, salt- and sugar-laden foods from their diets and replacing them with healthful whole foods, proponents of the Paleo diet have experienced myriad health benefits such as weight loss, better sleep, increased energy, and improvement or total reversal of many of the aforementioned diseases.

By eating a diet rich in wild game, fruits, vegetables, nuts, and seeds, Paleolithic man was able to avoid these modern ailments and do more than just survive his day-to-day life—he was able to thrive! For a more in-depth look at the history and science behind the Paleo diet, refer to *The Every-thing® Paleolithic Diet Book*, by Jodie and Gilaad Cohen.

What to Eat

Luckily, you don't have to spend all day hunting and gathering your food (unless, of course, you really want to), but you can still eat in much the same way that your ancestors did by consuming plenty of vegetables, fruits, protein, and healthy fats. These foods contain important vitamins, minerals, and antioxidants that work together to nourish your body and support your health in many different ways. For a complete list of Paleo pregnancy "yes" and "no" foods, refer to Appendix B at the end of this book.

Vegetables and Fruits

Vegetables and fruits are some of the most nutrient-dense sources of vitamins, minerals, fiber, and numerous phytonutrients. They are also your main source of carbohydrates on the Paleo diet. The more variety you include in your diet, the wider array of these important nutrients you will get. Some examples include:

- Apples
- Avocados
- Bananas
- Berries
- Cucumbers
- Dark leafy greens (broccoli, cabbage, Brussels sprouts, collard greens, kale, spinach, etc.)
- Melons
- Peppers
- Squash and zucchini
- Tomatoes

QUESTION

What are phytonutrients?
According to Douglas L. Margel's *The Nutrient-Dense Eating Plan*, phytonutrients are compounds that are responsible for the taste, smell, and pigment of plants, including fruits, vegetables, and herbs. They are not considered vital nutrients because they do not prevent specific diseases, but they do promote optimal health thanks to their protective properties, which range from protecting eye health to improving blood sugar regulation and providing anticancer benefits. Some well-known phytonutrients include beta carotene, carotenoids, flavonoids, and lycopene.

Animal Proteins

Animal proteins, including meat, seafood, and eggs, are optimal sources of nutrients that are essential for your body to function properly. Protein is made up of smaller building blocks called amino acids, and animal foods are the only foods considered to be complete proteins, meaning they contain all of the essential amino acids. Animal proteins also contain fats, which provide essential fatty acids (EFAs) that cannot be manufactured in your body and must be obtained from food sources. Some examples include:

- Eggs
- Fatty fish (mackerel, salmon, sardines, tuna, etc.)
- Lean fish (cod, halibut, tilapia, etc.)
- Poultry (chicken, duck, turkey, etc.)
- Red meat (beef, bison, lamb, pork, etc.)
- Shellfish (crab, oysters, scallops, shrimp, etc.)

Nuts and Seeds

Nuts and seeds are good dietary sources of fat and protein, but plant-based protein sources are not considered complete proteins, so be sure to include a variety of small amounts of nuts and seeds in your diet. Nuts and seeds also contain a blend of saturated, monounsaturated, and polyunsaturated fats, all of which are part of a healthy diet. Nuts can be consumed raw or made into nut butters or meal/flour. Some examples include:

- Almonds
- Almond meal/flour
- Cashew butter
- Hazelnuts
- Macadamia nuts
- Pecans
- Pumpkin seeds
- Sunflower seeds
- Walnuts

Fats and Oils

Luckily, the long-standing myths that criticize dietary fat have been dispelled. While any food eaten in excess is not going to be beneficial to your health, dietary fat is a vital and necessary part of any healthy eating plan. Fat provides more energy (calories) per gram than carbohydrates or protein and it also facilitates the absorption of the fat-soluble vitamins A, D, E, and K. The key is consuming healthy, naturally occurring fats and oils and striking a good balance between saturated and unsaturated fats and the essential omega-3 and omega-6 fatty acids. Good sources include:

- Avocado oil
- Coconut oil
- Extra virgin olive oil
- Flaxseed oil
- Ghee (clarified butter)
- Macadamia oil

ESSENTIAL

Omega-3 and omega-6 fatty acids are considered essential fatty acids because they must be consumed through your diet. Omega-6s are pro-inflammatory while omega-3s are anti-inflammatory. Inflammation is necessary to fight infection and injury, but chronic inflammation is the condition behind many modern diseases. Fatty fish, pastured beef, flaxseeds, and walnuts are good sources of omega-3 fatty acids.

A Note about Food Quality

On a Paleo diet, food quality is just as important as nutrient density. Organic fruits and vegetables are grown in healthy, nutrient-rich soil that is free of chemical pesticides and herbicides. According to Eatwild (*www .eatwild.com*), pastured meat and eggs have higher levels of omega-3 fatty acids and certain vitamins, are lower in calories and overall fat content, and do not contain the hormones, antibiotics, and other drugs that are often used in conventionally raised animals. In the same vein, wild-caught seafood has not been treated with antibiotics and is higher in protein and omega-3 fatty acids than farm-raised fish. Healthy food starts with healthy plants and animals!

Foods to Avoid

As you can see, all of the foods included in the Paleo diet are nutrient-dense and supportive of health. They were abundant prior to modern agriculture and factory farming. The foods that are not a part of the Paleo diet have been linked with many digestive disorders and modern diseases such as diabetes and cardiovascular disease. Some of the foods that you would avoid on the Paleo diet, such as fast food and candy, aren't even real food.

Grains

Grains were not a regular part of the human diet until about 10,000 years ago, which isn't long considering the millions of years hominids have been on Earth. Today grains make up a large part of the standard American diet, even though they contain high levels of anti-nutrients such as gluten, lectins, and phytic acid, and their micronutrient profiles pale in comparison to fruits and vegetables. On top of that, most of America's grain consumption is in the form of heavily refined products such as cereal, baked goods, and bread, which cause blood sugar spikes and crashes. Over time, a diet high in refined grains can lead to chronically elevated blood sugar levels and, eventually, type 2 diabetes. Some examples of grains that Americans consume in various forms, including as flours, include:

- Barley (gluten-containing grain)
- Corn
- Oats
- Rice
- Rye (gluten-containing grain)
- Wheat (gluten-containing grain)

QUESTION

What is an anti-nutrient?
Anti-nutrients are compounds that inhibit your ability to absorb the nutrients in your food and that can cause digestive distress, leading to serious disease over time. Lectins and gluten are proteins that can damage the lining of the small intestine, and phytic acid binds with minerals in food and prevent them from being absorbed. There are many anti-nutrients, but these three are found in high levels in grains, legumes, and refined foods.

Dairy

Not until the domestication of animals about 10,000 years ago did humans begin to consume dairy products as a part of their regular diet, making dairy another food group that has not been around all that long when you look at the big picture. Today, most commercial dairy comes from large factory farms that treat their animals with hormones and antibiotics, which are then passed to you through the milk. Commercial dairy products are also pasteurized and homogenized, which changes the molecular structure of the proteins and kills beneficial bacteria. Many people have trouble digesting milk products because of an allergy to the milk protein casein or the inability to digest lactose, the sugar found in milk. Milk is actually one of the most common food allergens, and the Genetics Home Reference website (*http://ghr.nlm.nih.gov*) reports that approximately 65 percent of the human population is lactose intolerant. Dairy includes milk and milk products from cows, goats, and sheep. Some examples include:

- Cheese
- Cottage cheese
- Milk
- Sour cream
- Yogurt

Beans and Legumes

Like grains, beans and legumes contain high levels of anti-nutrients in the form of lectins and phytic acid, and they are not nearly as good a source of protein as animal foods. Like other plant-based proteins, they are deficient in one or more of the essential amino acids. Note that this does not include snow peas, sugar snap peas, or green beans; because you are eating more pod than bean with these foods, the anti-nutrients are less concentrated and your body is better able to absorb the vitamins and minerals. Some examples of beans and legumes with high levels of anti-nutrients include:

- Black beans
- Garbanzo beans
- Lentils

- Peanuts (and peanut butter)
- Green peas
- Pinto beans
- Soy

Refined Sugar and Artificial Sweeteners

The naturally occurring sugar in fruit is completely different than the refined sugar found in most packaged snacks and cereals, baked goods, sweetened fruit juices, and sodas. Not only is refined sugar highly concentrated; it is also devoid of the fiber, water, vitamins, minerals, and phytonutrients that you get when you eat fruit. Your body has to actually pull from its own nutrient stores to metabolize refined sugar.

The simple carbohydrates in sugar have similar effects on your body as other refined carbohydrate foods: blood sugar spikes, mood swings, behavioral issues, obesity, diabetes, and other inflammatory diseases. Added sugars are often hidden under various names on food labels, but they are all detrimental to your health. Natural sweeteners such as honey, maple syrup, and molasses do provide some health benefits and are fine in moderation. Artificial sweeteners are man-made chemical compounds, certainly not something our ancestors would have eaten. Among other health issues, they have been linked with headaches, neurological disorders, digestive issues, and weight gain.

When reading food labels, look for the following words to clue you in that the food contains some form of refined or artificial sweetener:

- Anything ending in "-ose" (dextrose, sucrose, etc.)
- Anything ending in "-tol" (mannitol, sorbitol, or xylitol)
- Aspartame (Equal, NutraSweet)
- Juice
- Malt
- Saccharin (Sweet'N Low)
- Stevia
- Sucralose (Splenda)
- Syrup

Refined Foods and Fast Food

The more heavily a food is refined, the less nutrition it is going to provide. Fast food, cereals, baked goods, candy, chips, frozen meals, and even foods that are advertised as healthy (such as granola bars and crackers) go through a heavy refining process and usually contain a lot of ingredients. There are always exceptions, but you'll usually find refined sweeteners, hydrogenated (man-made, unnatural) fats, preservatives, MSG, and artificial flavors and/ or colors on the ingredients lists for these foods. Unless cold-pressed, seed oils such as canola and soybean oil also fall into the refined foods category, because the oils are chemically extracted from the seed—unlike olive oil or coconut oil, which can be extracted using natural methods.

ALERT

Certain processed foods, like sausage, salsa, nut butters, and certain snack bars, are great options on a Paleo diet as long as you read the ingredient labels carefully. When buying packaged foods or snacks, ask yourself the following questions: Is this food perishable? Does this food contain only a few ingredients that you can recognize and pronounce? Can you name the whole food(s) that this product was made from?

Healthy Diet = Healthy Mom and Baby

Now you've learned the benefits of eating certain foods and avoiding others on a Paleo diet, but you may be wondering how this diet applies to pregnancy. How do these foods support your health and the health of your growing baby? During pregnancy, your body is going through amazing changes: your uterus, breast tissue, and placenta are growing, your blood volume and flow are increasing, and your body is accumulating fat stores to nourish your baby. At the same time, your baby is experiencing rapid growth and development in the womb. All of these processes are supported by the nutrients you consume. Among other things, protein supports growth, healthy fats facilitate brain development, and carbohydrates provide both of you with the energy to make it all happen. Whole foods, such as those included in the Paleo diet, are the highest-quality, most nutrient-dense sources of these nutrients, as well as vitamins, minerals, and phytonutrients. For more information on the nutrients that are most important during pregnancy and how they support your health and the health of your baby, refer to Chapter 2. There may be no other time in your life when nutrition is as important as it is during pregnancy. A nourishing diet, along with regular exercise, low stress, and adequate rest, can have a tremendous impact on your pregnancy.

FACT

According to the American College of Obstetricians and Gynecologists (ACOG), a baby is considered full term when he is born between the thirty-ninth and fortieth week of pregnancy. Your baby is growing throughout pregnancy, all the way up to those important final weeks. Many of your baby's internal organs, including the brain, lungs, and liver, need the full term of pregnancy to fully develop.

None of this growth and development can take place without energy and nutrients from the food you eat. Because your body is working extra hard during pregnancy, your nutrient and energy requirements increase and it is more important than ever to consume high-quality, whole, Paleo foods. A healthy diet during pregnancy increases your chances of having a low-risk pregnancy and delivering a healthy, full-term baby.

Changing Nutritional Needs During Pregnancy

Even when you are resting, your energy expenditure increases during pregnancy because your heart and lungs are working harder to deliver nutrients and oxygen to your baby. This means you need extra calories every day— about 75,000 extra calories over the course of your pregnancy. You'll need about 100 extra calories per day in the first trimester, and 300 to 400 extra calories per day in the second and third trimesters. These numbers can vary if you are entering into pregnancy either underweight or overweight or if you are having multiples, so be sure to discuss your individual needs with your health care provider.

There is no need for you to start counting calories, though. Typically, you will get everything you need by taking a daily prenatal vitamin and eating the fresh, whole foods included in the Paleo diet. Try adding half of an avocado to your breakfast plate, drinking a refreshing coconut milk smoothie as a midmorning snack, or eating an apple and a handful of trail mix after dinner. Small additions like these will provide you with enough calories to meet your increasing energy needs.

ESSENTIAL

You can put endless combinations of Paleo foods on your plate, but there are a few general guidelines to follow to achieve a healthy balance. Fill half of your plate with vegetables and fruits and the rest with protein and healthy fats. While healthy fats can come in the form of avocado, nuts, or olives, they can also include the oil used to cook your vegetables or the oil in the dressing atop your salad, in which case they wouldn't have their own "spot" on your plate.

The key when it comes to pregnancy nutrition is variety and balance. You want to include a mix of carbohydrates, protein, and healthy fats at each meal so that you are getting enough of each, and the additional nutrients they provide, throughout the day. The more variety, the better, as each food on the Paleo diet provides different vitamins, minerals, and phytonutrients that work together to promote optimal health and well-being.

Planning Ahead for Paleo Success

You have probably heard the expression "failing to plan is planning to fail." This statement definitely holds true when it comes to pregnancy nutrition. Common pregnancy symptoms such as hunger, cravings, morning sickness (which should really be called "all-day sickness"), and food aversions can hit anytime, anywhere, so it is important to be prepared. Planning and preparation will help you to hold these symptoms at bay while sticking to your Paleo lifestyle.

Meal Planning

A great way to get started is with meal planning. Planning your meals for the coming week can help to ensure that you buy all of the groceries you need in one trip and that you'll always know what's on the menu, instead of staring blankly into the refrigerator after a long day at work. Building your grocery list based on your meal plan will also help you to avoid impulse purchases at the store. If you know you have a busy week coming up, consider making a large soup or chili in the slow cooker that you can easily reheat throughout the week.

Plan Your Snacks, Too

Speaking of impulses, it is equally important to be prepared with the right snacks when hunger strikes. Keep small snacks such as nuts and dried fruit in your purse or create a "snack drawer" at work with these items and other nonperishable foods such as jerky, tuna, and sun-dried tomatoes. If you have access to a refrigerator, you can also stock up on fresh fruit, organic and nitrate-free deli meats, veggie sticks, salsa, and guacamole. It's good to have a variety of foods on hand, because cravings and food aversions can be unpredictable and you never know what might sound good at any given time. Having the right snacks on hand can also help with morning sickness. For many women, having a small snack before getting out of bed in the morning and never going too long between meals can help to alleviate that queasy feeling.

Let this book serve as a guide and source of support throughout your pregnancy. With the right tools and a little nutrition knowledge, it is easier than you may think to stick to your Paleo lifestyle while nourishing your body and your growing baby.

CHAPTER 2

Health Benefits of a Paleo Pregnancy

Although pregnant women are often advised to drink milk for calcium and eat "heart-healthy" whole grains for vitamins, minerals, and fiber, these are not the only (or even the best) sources of the nutrients that are essential for you and your baby. If you are already following a Paleo diet, you can easily tailor it to your pregnancy. If you are new to the Paleo lifestyle but want to eat this way to care for your growing baby, this chapter will teach you which nutrients to focus on, why they're important, and how to get them.

The Vitamins, Minerals, and Healthy Fats You Need

You really can't go wrong when you are eating the fresh, wholesome foods on the Paleo diet, but during pregnancy there are certain nutrients that are crucial for your baby's development and for your own changing body. By filling up on nutrient-dense foods and avoiding cigarettes, alcohol and other drugs, you can decrease the risk of birth defects and pregnancy complications and also help to ensure your baby's health for years to come.

Following are the Recommended Dietary Allowances (RDAs) for the vitamins and minerals you need during pregnancy, and some further explanation of those that are most critical. These numbers are developed by the Food and Nutrition Board of the National Academy of Sciences' Institute of Medicine, and they provide a good general guideline. However, your needs may vary based on your age, weight, and other lifestyle factors, so be sure to talk with your health care provider about your individual recommendations. Recent research also shows that while these levels are high enough to prevent disease, they may not be high enough for optimal nutrition. You don't necessarily have to get the recommended amount each day, but make it your goal to reach or exceed the RDA as an average over a few days. It can be difficult to reach the daily intake of some of these nutrients through diet alone, but taking a high-quality daily prenatal vitamin can provide a little extra "insurance" that you'll be getting the nutrients you need. Discuss your need for a prenatal vitamin and other supplements with your health care provider.

RECOMMENDED DIETARY ALLOWANCES	
Calcium	1,000 mg (milligrams)
Choline	450 mg
Copper	1,000 mcg (micrograms)
DHA	600 mcg
Folate	600 mcg
Iodine	220 mcg
Iron	27 mg
Magnesium	350–360 mg
Niacin	18 mg

RECOMMENDED DIETARY ALLOWANCES	
Riboflavin	1.4 mg
Selenium	60 mcg
Thiamin	1.4 mg
Vitamin A	770 mcg
Vitamin B_6	1.9 mg
Vitamin B_{12}	2.6 mcg
Vitamin C	85 mg
Vitamin D	600 IU (International Units)
Vitamin E	15 mg
Vitamin K	90 mcg
Zinc	11 mg

Source: Food and Nutrition Board, Institute of Medicine, National Academies

Folate/Folic Acid

Folate is necessary for the production of red blood cells and the production, repair, and functioning of DNA. During pregnancy, when your body is rapidly producing new red blood cells for the placenta and for your baby, folate helps to prevent neural tube defects such as spina bifida and anencephaly. The Centers for Disease Control and Prevention report that women who consume the recommended daily dose of folate starting at least one month prior to conception and during the first trimester reduce their risk of these birth defects by 50 to 70 percent.

ALERT

Many people use the terms *folate* and *folic acid* interchangeably, but they are actually two different things. Folate, also known as vitamin B_9, is found naturally in foods such as liver, dark leafy greens, and citrus fruits, while folic acid is the synthetic form that is typically used in supplements, including many prenatal vitamins. Both provide the same protective benefits during pregnancy, so be sure to include a variety of folate-rich foods along with any supplements you and your health care provider choose to include.

The neural tube begins to form during the first few weeks of pregnancy, before many women even realize they are pregnant, so whether you are already pregnant or planning to become pregnant, it is a good idea to start increasing your folate intake now. Good sources of folate include:

- 3 ounces beef liver, 215 mcg
- ½ cup boiled spinach, 131 mcg
- 4 spears boiled asparagus, 89 mcg
- ½ cup boiled Brussels sprouts, 78 mcg
- ½ cup boiled broccoli, 52 mcg
- 1 small orange, 29 mcg
- 1 medium banana, 24 mcg

Source: National Institutes of Health, Office of Dietary Supplements

Calcium

Calcium is critical during pregnancy to help your baby form strong bones and teeth. To help you reach these higher levels, your body's ability to absorb calcium actually increases during pregnancy, and calcium loss (through your urine) decreases. If you do not consume enough calcium during pregnancy, your body will pull from its own calcium stores to provide for the baby, which could increase your risk of osteoporosis later in life.

Contrary to popular belief, you don't need to consume dairy to get calcium. Foods high in vitamin D, such as fatty fish and egg yolks, and foods high in magnesium, such as most dark leafy greens, nuts, and seeds, aid in calcium absorption. Good sources of calcium include:

- 3 ounces oil-canned sardines with bones, 325 mg
- 3 ounces canned pink salmon with bones, 181 mg
- ½ cup boiled turnip greens, 99 mg
- 1 cup chopped cooked kale, 94 mg
- 1 tablespoon sesame seeds, 88 mg
- 1 ounce dry roasted almonds, 75 mg
- 1 ounce dried figs, 45 mg

- 1 tablespoon blackstrap molasses, 41 mg
- 1 cup raw broccoli, 42 mg

Sources: National Institutes of Health, Office of Dietary Supplements; Self Nutrition Data (http://nutritiondata.self.com)

Iron

During pregnancy, blood volume and circulation increase to support the growth of the placenta and to nourish your baby. Iron is necessary for the production of red blood cells, and adequate intake decreases your risk of anemia, which can lead to complications such as preterm birth and low birth weight. If you are exhibiting signs of anemia, your health care provider will most likely perform a blood test to check your iron levels and may recommend supplementation. Foods rich in vitamin C, including dark leafy greens and citrus fruits, help to increase iron absorption, so it is a good idea to eat these foods together. Good sources of iron include:

- 3 ounces beef liver, 5 mg
- 3 ounces ground beef, 2.2 mg
- 3 ounces canned sardines with bones, 2 mg
- 1 ounce pumpkin seeds, 4.2 mg
- 1 tablespoon blackstrap molasses, 3.5 mg
- ½ cup boiled spinach, 3 mg
- 1 ounce roasted cashews, 2 mg
- ¼ cup raisins, 1 mg

Sources: National Institutes of Health, Office of Dietary Supplements; Centers for Disease Control and Prevention

FACT

Heme, the form of iron that comes from animal sources, is more bioavailable than the non-heme iron found in plant sources, so be sure to consume a variety of iron-rich plant and animal foods to meet your daily iron requirements.

Trace Minerals

Trace minerals are needed in much smaller amounts than other minerals, usually less than 15 milligrams per day, but they still play a significant role in the health of you and your baby during pregnancy. Iodine, found mostly in seafood and sea vegetables, supports thyroid regulation and brain and nervous system development. Copper, found in shellfish, nuts, and seeds, is involved in the formation of the heart, blood vessels, and skeletal and nervous systems. Zinc, found in red meat, shellfish, poultry, nuts, and seeds, is necessary for the production, function, and repair of DNA, which is essential during the rapid cell growth that takes place during pregnancy. Because these minerals are needed in such small amounts, supplementation is not usually necessary.

Vitamin C

Vitamin C holds many benefits outside of its role in helping with iron absorption. Vitamin C is necessary for the formation of collagen, a structural component of cartilage, tendons, bones, and skin. Good sources include:

- ½ cup raw sweet red pepper, 95 mg
- 1 medium orange, 70 mg
- ½ cup cooked broccoli, 51 mg
- ½ cup fresh sliced strawberries, 49 mg
- ½ cup cooked Brussels sprouts, 48 mg
- ½ cup cooked cabbage, 28 mg
- ½ cup raw cauliflower, 26 mg

Source: National Institutes of Health, Office of Dietary Supplements

Vitamin B_6

Because vitamin B_6 plays a part in the production of red blood cells, it is vital for your baby's brain and nervous system development. Only a small amount is needed each day, so it is easy to reach your daily intake through diet alone.

Good sources of vitamin B_6 include:

- 3 ounces beef liver, .9 mg
- 3 ounces cooked yellowfin tuna, .9 mg
- 3 ounces roasted chicken breast, .6 mg
- 1 medium banana, .4 mg
- 3 ounces ground beef, .3 mg
- ½ cup baked winter squash, .2 mg
- 1 ounce mixed nuts, .1 mg

Source: National Institutes of Health, Office of Dietary Supplements

ESSENTIAL

Morning sickness got you down? Current research findings, including a 2009 study in the *Midwifery* journal, show that vitamin B_6 may help to alleviate nausea and vomiting during pregnancy. Consult with your health care provider before taking supplemental B_6.

Vitamin D

Vitamin D is required for your body to properly absorb calcium, and, as you'll recall, calcium helps to build your baby's strong bones and teeth. According to the World Health Organization, proper vitamin D levels may also promote healthy birth weight and decrease your risk of gestational diabetes, preeclampsia, and preterm birth. Vitamin D is not naturally occurring in many foods, but your body can manufacture vitamin D through exposure to sunlight. Because most people do not spend enough time outside or consume enough vitamin D–rich foods, vitamin D deficiency is common, and many researchers are now recommending that pregnant women get much higher levels than the current RDA. High-quality supplements, such as cod liver oil, are safe and widely available, so ask your health care provider to test your vitamin D levels to determine your individual needs. Good sources include:

- 1 tablespoon cod liver oil, 1,360 IU (International Units)
- 3 ounces cooked salmon, 447 IU

- 3 ounces canned tuna, 154 IU
- 3 ounces beef liver, 42 IU
- 2 sardines, 46 IU
- 1 large egg (vitamin D is found in the yolk), 41 IU

Source: National Institutes of Health, Office of Dietary Supplements

ALERT

While liver contains high levels of many of the nutrients you need during pregnancy, too much liver may actually be problematic. Liver contains high amounts of preformed vitamin A, or retinol. Some research suggests that too much retinol, especially early in pregnancy, has been linked with birth defects. There is no reason to avoid liver entirely as long as you enjoy it in moderation with a variety of other healthy Paleo foods.

Water

Water is not a vitamin or mineral, but it does transport these elements to your blood cells, and those blood cells then travel to the placenta to nourish your baby. Water is necessary to support fetal circulation, amniotic fluid levels, and your increasing blood volume during pregnancy. Water also flushes toxins out of your body, promotes healthy digestion, and can help ease common pregnancy symptoms such as fatigue, headaches, dry skin, bloating, constipation, and swelling.

QUESTION

How much water do I need during pregnancy?
Aim for at least eight (8-ounce) glasses of drinking water each day. You'll want extra water before, during, and after exercise. You can get additional water by eating plenty of fruits and vegetables and drinking tea, broth, and 100 percent fruit or vegetable juices.

Benefits of Omega-3 Fatty Acids

Omega-3 fatty acids are essential fatty acids (EFAs) that are necessary for the development of your baby's brain, retina, immune system, and central nervous system, as well as the production of adrenal and sex hormones. Omega-3s are considered "essential" because they cannot be made in the body, so you must consume them either through your diet or in a fish oil supplement. As outlined in *Reviews in Obstetrics & Gynecology*, studies have shown higher scores on IQ tests in children whose mothers had higher EFA levels through seafood consumption during pregnancy. EFA consumption may also decrease your risk of preeclampsia, preterm birth, and postpartum depression. Good sources of omega-3s include:

- Dark leafy greens (broccoli, cabbage, Brussels sprouts, collard greens, kale, spinach, etc.)
- Fish oil supplement
- Flaxseed (and flaxseed oil)
- Salmon
- Sardines
- Shrimp
- Tuna
- Walnuts

ALERT

Pregnant women are warned to limit fish intake due to the high mercury levels found in some fish. In high doses, mercury is dangerous to the development of your baby's brain and nervous system. To lessen this risk, look for high-quality sources of wild-caught seafood, and aim for 1–2 servings per week. Because of high mercury levels, it is best to avoid shark, swordfish, king mackerel, and tilefish during pregnancy. Better choices include salmon, tilapia, anchovies, sardines, ocean perch, and shellfish, which are among the lowest in mercury. Mercury levels in large fish such as tuna can vary, though canned, light tuna has been found to have lower levels than albacore or yellowfin.

Balancing Blood Sugar Levels

Hormonal changes during pregnancy can cause your body to become less responsive to insulin, triggering blood sugar levels to rise higher than usual. During pregnancy, maintaining balanced blood sugar levels decreases your risk of certain complications, including gestational diabetes and preeclampsia. It also decreases the chance that your baby will be born with a high birth weight, which can make for a difficult delivery and has even been linked with obesity into childhood and adulthood. Balanced blood sugar levels can even ease common pregnancy symptoms such as morning sickness, cravings, and mood swings.

By following a Paleo diet during pregnancy, you are naturally removing the refined carbohydrates and highly sweetened foods and beverages that cause the blood sugar spikes and crashes that contribute to insulin resistance. A diet full of fiber-rich fruits and vegetables and hunger-satisfying protein and fats can go a long way toward maintaining proper blood sugar. Consider the following tips for maintaining balanced blood sugar during pregnancy:

- Increase fiber and complex carbohydrate intake from fresh fruits and vegetables.
- Consume adequate protein and healthy fats so you always feel satiated.
- Don't go longer than three to four hours without eating.
- Eat breakfast within an hour of waking up.
- If you need to, have a small snack when you wake up or just before bed.
- Carry snacks in your purse, your gym bag, even your glove box. And always keep your home and office well stocked.
- Plan meals and snacks ahead of time (as outlined in Chapter 1).

Organic Fruits and Vegetables

Organic fruits and vegetables are free of herbicides, pesticides, and fertilizers that may pose a variety of health risks to you and your baby. The "Dirty Dozen" are the fruits and vegetables that are found to have the highest levels of pesticide residue. This list is put together by the Environmental Working

Group (*www.ewg.org/foodnews*) and is updated annually. If you can only allocate a portion of your budget toward organic produce, try to purchase organic varieties of these fruits and vegetables to minimize your exposure to pesticide residues. The current list includes:

- Apples
- Strawberries
- Grapes
- Celery
- Peaches
- Spinach
- Sweet Bell Peppers
- Nectarines (imported)
- Cucumbers
- Cherry Tomatoes
- Snap Peas (imported)
- Potatoes

Source: Environmental Working Group, 2014

As an added benefit, organic fruits and vegetables are higher in nutrients because they are grown in mineral-rich, chemically untreated soil that is often fertilized with organic matter, such as food scraps, leaves, and plants. A 2010 study published in the *Alternative Medicine Review* found that many organically grown foods were higher in vitamin C, iron, magnesium, phosphorus, and phytonutrients.

ESSENTIAL

Take your organic shopping one step further and go for a weekend walk to your neighborhood farmers' market. Not all produce at the farmers' market is grown organically, but organic growers will usually have signage letting you know that their produce is free of chemicals. Even better, by shopping at the farmers' market, you are supporting local producers and ensuring that you and your baby are getting the freshest and most highly nutritious fruits and vegetables available.

Grass-Fed and Free-Range Proteins

Chickens and pigs were meant to root around for bugs and seeds, and cows were meant to eat grass. They were not meant to live on feedlots or in cages and fed genetically modified grains and soy. When you buy meat and eggs labeled as grass-fed and free-range or pasture-raised, you know that the animals were raised humanely and fed a natural diet. For a farm to receive the American Grassfed Association's seal of approval, its animals must be fed only grass and forage, must be raised without confinement to feedlots, and must never be treated with antibiotics or growth hormones.

Not only are pastured meat and eggs safer, they are also higher in certain nutrients. As mentioned in Chapter 1, according to Eatwild (*www.eatwild.com*), pastured meat and eggs have higher levels of omega-3s and certain vitamins and are lower in calories and overall fat content than conventionally raised animals. Wild-caught seafood is safer for you and your baby as well: it is raised on a natural diet, has not been treated with antibiotics, and is higher in protein and omega-3s than farm-raised fish.

Pastured meat and eggs and wild-caught seafood will always be labeled accordingly. Many conventional grocery stores are beginning to carry these products, and they are also widely available at health food stores, farmers' markets, butcher shops, local farms, and even online. When animals are healthy, you know the food you are eating is healthy too.

Selecting the Best Superfoods

All foods included in the Paleo diet are nutrient-dense, but there are some standout superfoods at the top of the list that provide the highest levels of the vitamins, minerals, and healthy fats you need during pregnancy. Following is a list of some of the top pregnancy foods that will get you the most bang for your nutritional buck.

PREGNANCY SUPERFOODS	
Food	Nutrients
Avocado	Fiber, folate, omega-3 fatty acids, vitamin C, vitamin K
Beef	Choline, iron, niacin, protein, selenium, vitamin B_6, vitamin B_{12}, zinc
Berries	Vitamin C, fiber, folate, phytonutrients
Broccoli	Calcium, fiber, folate, phytonutrients, riboflavin, vitamin A, vitamin B_6, vitamin C, vitamin E, vitamin K
Dark leafy greens	Calcium, fiber, folate, iron, phytonutrients, vitamin A, vitamin C, vitamin K
Eggs	Choline, iodine, iron, protein, riboflavin, selenium, vitamin B_{12}
Salmon	Calcium, niacin, omega-3 fatty acids, protein, selenium, vitamin B_6, vitamin B_{12}, vitamin D
Sweet potatoes	Fiber, folate, phytonutrients, vitamin A, vitamin C
Walnuts	Copper, magnesium, omega-3 fatty acids, protein, vitamin B_6, zinc

Source: Self Nutrition Data (http://nutritiondata.self.com)

Need a few ideas to get you started? You can make these superfoods even more super by combining them with these simple, tasty meal and snack ideas:

- Garden Veggie Omelet (see Chapter 7)
- Garlic Broccoli and Beef (see Chapter 9)
- Salmon Muffins (see Chapter 11)
- Baked Sweet Potato Fries (see Chapter 12)
- California Salad (see Chapter 13)

CHAPTER 3

Practical Considerations

Pregnancy is a miraculous, life-changing journey. You may be overflowing with that blissed-out pregnancy glow, but you are most likely overflowing with questions and concerns as well. "How do I find the right doctor? How can I make it through the day with fatigue and morning sickness? Is it safe to eat my favorite foods? What do I do when cravings hit in the middle of the night?" Pregnancy can be a fun, exciting, and enjoyable time as long as you know how to navigate some of these common issues.

Finding a Health Care Provider

Finding the right health care provider is one of the first things you should do when you discover you are pregnant. You'll be seeing a lot of him or her over the next nine months, so it is important to shop around for someone you are compatible with. You will have to make a lot of decisions regarding pregnancy, labor, and delivery; you'll want to choose someone who can guide and inform you, but ultimately support your choices as a mother-to-be.

Prenatal Care Provider Options

You may already have a doctor or midwife whom you want to continue seeing during your pregnancy. If not, you have a few options to choose from. There are different types of prenatal care practitioners, each with different specialties and areas of expertise. Here is a brief rundown of your choices:

- **Family physician:** A family physician is a primary doctor with the well-rounded training to care for people in all stages of life, including pregnancy and childbirth. If your pregnancy is relatively low risk, this can be a great option—you can continue your relationship with her after you give birth, and she can even become your baby's pediatric health care provider.
- **Obstetrician-Gynecologist (Ob-Gyn):** An ob-gyn is a medical doctor who specializes in female reproductive health, prenatal care, childbirth, and postpartum care. Ob-gyns are also trained in surgery and are able to perform C-section deliveries.
- **Maternal-fetal medicine specialist:** If you have health problems or are at risk for pregnancy complications, your health care provider may refer you to a maternal-fetal medicine specialist; these providers have extensive training in high-risk pregnancies.
- **Midwife:** Midwives have professional training in all aspects of female health and wellness, including pregnancy, labor and delivery, and the postpartum period. Many midwives are also registered nurses. If your pregnancy is low risk and you are planning an unmedicated delivery, you may choose to see a midwife. Depending on your location, midwives can deliver in hospitals, birthing centers, or your home.

- **Prenatal provider team:** Many providers work with a team of other doctors, midwives, and nurse practitioners. You may see the midwives or nurse practitioners if your pregnancy is low-risk and only see the doctor if complications arise. When it is time to deliver your baby, you will most likely see the on-call provider, so it is a good idea to meet with various members of the team throughout your pregnancy so you can get to know each of them.

QUESTION

What is a doula?
While they cannot provide routine prenatal care, doulas are practitioners who can provide emotional and physical support during pregnancy, childbirth, and beyond. Among other things, a doula can help you develop a birth plan, attend your birth and help you cope with labor pains naturally, help prepare your home for a newborn, assist you with breastfeeding, and even stock your kitchen with healthy meals.

Where to Search

It is understandable that you want to find just the right person to care for you during pregnancy. Your prenatal care provider will be a big part of your life in the coming months, and you should look for someone you are comfortable with and whom you trust. With so many providers to choose from, though, how do you decide on the right one for you? Here are a few tips to help you narrow down the search:

- **Friends and family:** Friends and family members are a great resource for health care provider recommendations, especially if their pregnancy and birth experience was similar to the one you are hoping for.
- **Ask your doctor:** If your family doctor does not offer prenatal care, she should be able to suggest a practitioner to you.
- **Check with your insurance company:** Your insurance company may only provide coverage for certain practitioners in your area. They should be able to provide you with a list of in-network providers.

- **Call your preferred hospital or birthing center:** If there is a certain hospital or birthing center where you would like to deliver, give them a call to find out which doctors and midwives will deliver there.
- **Go online:** Still stumped? Take your search to the Internet. If you are searching for an ob-gyn, try the American Congress of Obstetricians and Gynecologists website (*www.acog.org*) and click on "Find an Ob-Gyn." To find a midwife in your area, visit the American College of Nurse-Midwives (*www.midwife.org*) and click on "Find a midwife."

Questions to Ask Potential Providers

Once you choose a health care provider, you'll want to make sure he is on board with your preferences for pregnancy, labor, and delivery. A quick look at the provider's website or a call to the office staff should answer many of your questions, or you can discuss your concerns at your first appointment. Some questions to keep in mind:

- Do they accept your insurance?
- What are the costs and payment options?
- Is the office location convenient to your home and/or work?
- Where will you deliver your baby?
- What is the procedure if they determine your pregnancy is high-risk?
- Who will you see at your regular prenatal visits?
- How do they handle after-hours phone calls?
- Who will deliver your baby?
- Will they help you determine a birth plan?
- What is their stance on and rate of medical interventions (induction, epidural, C-section, etc.)?
- Do they support the type of labor and birth you desire (unmedicated birth, ability to labor in the tub, etc.)?
- Are they familiar with the Paleo diet and will they be supportive of your choice to follow a Paleo diet during pregnancy?

At the end of the appointment, take some time to think about how you felt while talking with the practitioner. Did the practitioner explain what he was doing and why? Did you have to wait long and feel rushed through your appointment, or did you feel respected and that your questions were answered thoroughly? A good care provider will take the time to educate you and make you feel at ease. And remember, if things don't work out, you can switch providers at any time during your pregnancy.

ESSENTIAL

Childbirth education classes can ease some of the anxiety you may be feeling about pregnancy, labor, and delivery. You'll learn about the signs and stages of labor, pain relief options, and ways your partner can help, and you'll have the opportunity to bond with other moms-to-be. Check with your health care provider, other moms, or a local hospital or birthing center to find classes in your area.

Prenatal Vitamins and Supplements

There are varying schools of thought in the Paleo world on the need for prenatal vitamins. On one hand, some will argue that by eating a healthy Paleo diet you are getting all of the nutrients you and your baby need. Others feel that it isn't worth the risk that even a carefully planned diet may not be sufficient to provide your baby with everything required for proper growth and development. Because most people aren't going to take the time to calculate their daily calorie and nutrient intake, a prenatal vitamin can help to ensure that your bases are covered, especially if you are experiencing morning sickness and literally can't keep your food down. Any good prenatal vitamin should contain folate/folic acid, calcium, copper, iron, magnesium, zinc, vitamins A, C, D, E, and K, and the B vitamins (most vitamin supplements contain other vitamins and minerals, too). Some prenatal vitamins now contain DHA, as well. If yours doesn't, you can add in a daily dose of cod liver oil. The Mayo Clinic advises that prenatal vitamins should contain at least the following:

- Folic acid: 400 to 800 mcg (micrograms)
- Calcium: 250 mg (milligrams)
- Iron: 30 mg
- Vitamin C: 50 mg
- Zinc: 15 mg

- Copper: 2 mg
- Vitamin B_6: 2 mg
- Vitamin D: 400 IU (International Units)

What is DHA?
DHA, short for docosahexaenoic acid, is an omega-3 fatty acid that supports brain, eye, and nervous system health. During pregnancy and infancy, DHA is necessary for proper retinal and cognitive development. DHA cannot be produced in the body, but it is naturally occurring in breast milk and fatty fish or can be obtained through supplementation.

All prenatal vitamins are not created equal, though. Some vitamins contain artificial dyes and other additives. These have not been shown to have any negative effects on pregnancy, but you do have the option of seeking out vitamins that do not contain these ingredients. There are also vitamins available that use food-based (instead of synthetic) nutrients and contain digestive enzymes to increase absorption. The choice of vitamin is a decision that deserves careful thought and consideration and that should also be discussed with your health care provider. She may recommend other supplements, as well, depending on the specific ingredients in the prenatal vitamin you choose, your pre-pregnancy nutrient levels, or as a response to certain complications that may arise, such as severe morning sickness or iron deficiency.

If you are having trouble swallowing your prenatal vitamin or keeping it down because of morning sickness, try taking it with a small snack or in the evening just before going to bed. If this doesn't work, discuss the option of switching brands with your health care provider.

Foods and Substances to Avoid

During pregnancy, your immune system is suppressed because of hormonal changes in your body. This can make it harder to fight off infections, putting you at an increased risk for certain foodborne illnesses, such as salmonella, toxoplasmosis, and listeriosis, that can cause serious health problems for you and your baby. Safe food-handling practices such as washing surfaces and utensils, heating food thoroughly, washing your hands when preparing food, rinsing fruits and vegetables, and storing food properly can all help to lessen this risk, but there are also foods that are best avoided during pregnancy to further reduce your risk. These include undercooked meat and eggs, processed meats like deli meats and hot dogs (which should be cooked thoroughly before eating), and raw or smoked seafood.

You should also avoid alcohol, nicotine, and recreational drugs. Some herbs and herbal teas may not be safe during pregnancy, and even certain over-the-counter and prescription medications can be dangerous during pregnancy. There is also research that links caffeine intake during pregnancy with certain complications, such as low birth weight. Until there is conclusive evidence on the association between caffeine intake and its effect on pregnancy, the March of Dimes states that pregnant women should limit caffeine intake to no more than 200 milligrams per day. This is the equivalent of just one 12-ounce cup of coffee. Tea, soft drinks, chocolate, and certain medications and herbal supplements can contain caffeine as well, and need to be considered in your daily total intake.

Many of these recommendations are made in an abundance of caution because not enough is known about the effects of certain foods, medications, and other substances during pregnancy. Pregnant women are not included in medical and nutritional studies because of the possible danger to the mother and the baby. Discuss any and all herbs or medications with your health care provider before taking them.

Decreasing Your Risk of Common Pregnancy Complications

What you choose to eat during pregnancy can lower your risk for many dangerous complications. It isn't just the nutrients you take in, but also the type and amount of food you eat. Adequate weight gain, rest, regular exercise, and a Paleo diet will provide you with a solid nutritional base and help to lower your risk of certain complications and increase the chance that your baby will be born at full term with a healthy weight.

Low Birth Weight and Preterm Birth

Babies can be born with a low birth weight either because they are born prematurely (before 37 weeks) or because they experience slow growth in utero. Together, these are the leading causes of infant mortality. Low-birth-weight and preterm babies have a greater risk of complications throughout life because their organs may not be fully formed at birth. There are many factors that contribute to low birth weight and preterm birth, including any chronic health conditions you may have, infections that you or your baby contract during pregnancy, and certain birth defects, but eating a healthy diet and getting enough calories, avoiding drugs, alcohol, and nicotine, and routine prenatal care will greatly increase your chances of carrying your baby to term and delivering a healthy baby.

High Birth Weight

Babies whose weight is above the 90th percentile are considered large for gestational age and may experience problems during delivery, throughout childhood, and into adulthood. High-birth-weight babies are at greater risk for feeding problems, hypoglycemia, lung problems, and birth injuries to the shoulders and collarbone. Because of the risk of birth injuries, C-section delivery may be necessary. The National Institutes of Health reports that high-birth-weight babies also have a higher risk of obesity, asthma, and diabetes later in life. Managing your weight gain during pregnancy by staying active and following a nutritious Paleo diet will help to ensure that your baby is born at a healthy weight.

Gestational Diabetes

With the hormonal changes of pregnancy, your cells can become less responsive to insulin, which triggers a rise in blood glucose levels. If your body is not able to produce enough insulin to regulate your blood sugar levels, you are said to have gestational diabetes. Because the glucose in your blood is transferred to your baby's blood through the placenta, poorly managed gestational diabetes may cause your baby to be born with a high birth weight and the complications that come along with it.

Entering pregnancy at a healthy weight and sustaining proper weight gain during pregnancy can lessen your risk of developing gestational diabetes and help to manage blood sugar levels if you are diagnosed. When following a Paleo diet, you are already naturally avoiding the foods that cause blood glucose levels to rise quickly, such as refined sugars and carbohydrates, and you'll be filling up on complex carbohydrates and fiber from fruits and vegetables, both of which help your body to maintain normal blood sugar levels. Following the blood sugar–balancing tips in Chapter 2 will also help to keep your levels in check.

ALERT

Did you know that gestational diabetes actually increases your risk of developing type 2 diabetes later in life, and that women with gestational diabetes also have higher instances of preeclampsia?

You will most likely be tested for gestational diabetes between twenty-four and twenty-eight weeks, and you have some options here, as well. Many women on the Paleo diet do not want to consume the sugar-sweetened beverage (which also contains artificial dyes and flavors) that is most often used to perform the test, and if you are already following a Paleo diet and not normally consuming much sugar on a daily basis, the test could produce a false positive result. If this is a concern for you, talk with your health care provider about alternatives, such as keeping a food log and monitoring your blood sugar throughout the day using a glucometer or taking the test using real food options such as fruit or fruit juice.

Preeclampsia

Preeclampsia, also referred to as pregnancy-induced hypertension or toxemia of pregnancy, is a condition that can develop as the pregnancy advances, usually in the third trimester. It is characterized by high blood pressure, sudden swelling, and weight gain due to fluid retention and protein in urine. If well managed through monitoring by your care provider, limited physical activity, and plenty of rest, most mothers go on to deliver perfectly healthy babies. According to the Preeclampsia Foundation, there are many risk factors for preeclampsia, including obesity and diabetes. The World Health Organization (WHO) has published evidence that micronutrient deficiencies, especially calcium, may increase the risk of developing preeclampsia. This is just another reason why it is important to maintain a healthy weight and eat a nutritious diet before and during pregnancy.

Coping with Morning Sickness

The technical, and much more accurate, term for morning sickness is "nausea and vomiting of pregnancy." Morning sickness implies that you only experience this symptom in the morning, but most mothers will tell you that it can hit at any time. It is true that many women experience more severe symptoms in the morning that ease up as the day goes on, but others suffer from morning until night. Morning sickness can come and go throughout pregnancy and varies in intensity, but it is most common in the first trimester and usually subsides early in the second trimester.

QUESTION

What is hyperemesis gravidarum?
Hyperemesis gravidarum is excessive vomiting during pregnancy, a condition that affects only a small percentage of women. The condition should be promptly treated so that it does not cause any harm to you or your baby through dehydration or malnutrition. Talk with your health care provider if you have severe nausea and vomiting that does not subside after the first trimester, causes dehydration, leads to weight loss, or if you are unable to keep any food or liquid down.

Doctors have yet to determine exactly what causes morning sickness, but common theories include rapidly increasing hormone levels, heightened sense of smell, and even a defense mechanism to protect you from eating foods that may be dangerous to your baby. Whatever the cause, there are numerous remedies and treatments that may offer you some relief.

- **Eat before getting out of bed:** Eating a small snack before you get up and get moving can help to ease symptoms.

- **Eat small, frequent meals:** Because low blood sugar can contribute to that feeling of queasiness, eating small meals throughout the day ensures that you are never operating on an empty stomach.

- **Stay hydrated:** Dehydration can contribute to nausea and drinking water may keep that "empty stomach" feeling at bay. And if you are vomiting, you need extra water to replace lost fluids. If water doesn't sound appetizing, try adding a lemon or lime wedge or a sprig of fresh mint.

- **Ginger:** Some women find that ginger helps to settle their queasiness. Try adding powdered ginger to your smoothie or grate fresh ginger into hot water to make a ginger tea. If these don't help, discuss the option of taking a natural gingerroot supplement with your health care provider.

- **Have a variety of foods available:** What sounds good one morning may turn your stomach the next, so have a variety of foods available at home, work, and everywhere in between!

- **Vitamin B_6:** As mentioned in Chapter 2, vitamin B_6 has been shown to alleviate feelings of nausea during pregnancy. If nothing seems to be working, talk with your health care provider about supplemental vitamin B_6.

- **Eat what you can:** Don't worry if you can no longer stomach your favorite salad or can't stand to be in the same room as bacon frying in the pan. For now, eat what sounds good (even if that means eating the same foods day in and day out) and don't force yourself to eat anything that makes you feel nauseated. Morning sickness will pass and you will once again be able to eat a variety of healthy foods.

- **Take your prenatal vitamin later in the day:** If your symptoms are worse in the morning, don't take your prenatal vitamin on an empty stomach. Try taking your prenatal vitamin with breakfast or right before bed. If this doesn't help, discuss the option of switching prenatal vitamins with your health care provider. You may be sensitive to a particular brand of vitamins, but feel just fine when you switch to another.

- **Acupressure wristbands:** Available at most mass retailers and drugstores, these bands are usually intended for seasickness and motion sickness, but they may bring comfort during pregnancy as well.

- **Aromatherapy:** Certain scents, such as lemon, orange, or mint, have been shown to calm morning sickness for some women. You can use essential oils or the real thing.
- **Medication:** If you've exhausted all of your options (and are feeling pretty exhausted yourself), talk with your health care provider about anti-nausea medications that are safe during pregnancy.

Stabilizing Mood Swings

Mood swings during pregnancy are fairly common, and with good reason. Not only are your hormones raging, but your body is changing, you might be fatigued, and you are probably feeling a lot of new emotions trying to prepare for a baby. Take a deep breath; you are not alone, and there are even a few things you can do to enjoy some much needed peace of mind.

- **Exercise:** Exercise helps to boost your mood in more ways than one. Exercise produces endorphins, "feel-good" neurotransmitters released from the central nervous system and the pituitary gland that can keep your spirits high long after your workout is complete. Exercise can also boost your energy, help you sleep better, stretch your muscles, and reduce pain, swelling, and discomfort, all of which can help to keep a smile on your face. Try out a prenatal yoga class, go for a walk, or hit the gym for your favorite workout. For more information on exercise during pregnancy, including which exercises are safe and which to avoid, turn to Chapter 5.
- **Stress reduction:** Rest and relaxation are just as important as regular physical activity during pregnancy because your body is working extra hard to grow and nurture your baby. Now is a great time to put your feet up, remove added stress from your life, and get plenty of sleep as you prepare for the arrival of your little bundle of joy. Stress not only negatively influences your mood, it can also cause headaches, affect your appetite, suppress immune function, and contribute to high blood pressure, which can result in health problems for you and your baby. Read a book, take a nap, go for a walk, turn on your favorite music, write in a pregnancy journal, take a prenatal yoga class, take a bath, or do any other activity you find relaxing. If you are feeling anxious about labor

and delivery, sign up for a childbirth education class. Let friends and family lend a hand by helping to cook healthy meals, paint the nursery, or shop for baby necessities.

- **Eat well and often:** Low blood sugar can leave you feeling tired, anxious, and weak (not to mention hungry), and worsen morning sickness. Keep your blood sugar steady by having small meals and snacks throughout the day. Try to include fiber, protein, and fat in each meal, such as a spinach salad with blueberries, salmon, and avocado.

- **Talk it out:** If you are feeling down, talk with your partner or another mom who has been just where you are now. It can help to confide in someone, and it is reassuring to know that what you are feeling is a perfectly normal part of pregnancy.

Mood swings are usually most intense in the first trimester when hormone levels are highest, but can occur at any time during pregnancy. If your mood swings are frequent, intense, or last for more than a few weeks, talk with your practitioner. She can offer a variety of coping techniques or, if necessary, refer you to a counselor.

Dealing with Cravings

If you followed a Paleo diet for a while before getting pregnant, you may be taken by surprise when the freezer case of ice cream at the market starts calling your name or you wake in the middle of the night with visions of cheeseburgers dancing in your head. Strong food cravings are a typical pregnancy symptom that are, unfortunately, a bit of a mystery in the medical world. Some professionals attribute it to changing hormones, but others believe that it is your body's way of crying out for missing nutrients. Either way, cravings can be hard to ignore—but there are ways to combat your cravings while still sticking to your Paleo diet.

- **Stop cravings before they appear:** As with many other pregnancy symptoms, maintaining balanced blood sugar and never letting yourself get too hungry can also help stop cravings in their tracks. Always eat breakfast, and continue to eat small, frequent meals and snacks throughout the day.

- **Mix it up:** Keep a variety of fruits, vegetables, protein sources, and nutritious snacks on hand. When cravings and aversions are running rampant, you never know what might sound good at any given moment (and it may change from one meal to the next). By keeping your kitchen stocked with healthy options, you'll be ready when cravings strike.
- **Get creative:** Craving French fries? Try Baked Sweet Potato Fries (see Chapter 12) instead. Dreaming of chocolate? A batch of No-Bake Brownie Bites (see Chapter 16) will hit the spot! When a craving hits, take a moment to think about healthy substitutes that will keep you on track and allow you to indulge. For even more ideas, check out the Paleo recipes in Chapters 7 through 19.
- **Distraction:** Often, cravings will subside after only a few minutes. Try going for a short walk or calling up a friend and your cravings may melt away.
- **Remember why you are eating this way:** Remember why you are following a Paleo way of living in the first place: to provide your baby with essential nourishment for proper growth and development. You are in control of what goes into your body and what doesn't. Staying mindful of this can help keep you on track and making healthy choices.

QUESTION

What is pica?

The NIH defines pica as "a pattern of eating non-food materials, such as dirt or paper." In pregnancy, it is often attributed to iron and zinc deficiency. If you find yourself craving dirt, ice, sand, or other non-food items, speak with your health care provider immediately. Consuming non-food items can be extremely dangerous for both you and your unborn baby.

Food and Water Aversion

Aversions are just as mysterious and tricky as cravings, and can be just as strong. This is one of the first pregnancy symptoms you may experience, again most likely due to rapidly rising hormone levels. Aversions should taper off as you approach the second trimester, but certain aversions may stick with you throughout your entire pregnancy.

Especially in the early days when aversions are strongest, try to eat what you can and don't bother with foods that sound unappetizing. Even if you don't have the variety you typically enjoy in your diet, eating something is better than eating nothing. You'll have plenty of time in the second and third trimesters to dig back into your favorite foods. In the meantime, rely on your prenatal vitamins to make up for any nutrients that are lacking because the sight of broccoli or the smell of fish makes you sick. If the thought of downing eight glasses of water each day sounds impossible, try adding fruit slices or mint to your water, or try adding water to a fruit smoothie. You can also get more water in your diet by eating fruits and vegetables with high water content like cucumbers, tomatoes, peppers, strawberries, and watermelon.

What about Dairy?

Even outside of pregnancy, avoiding dairy is one of the most controversial aspects of the Paleo diet. With the prevalence of dairy allergies and intolerances and the hormones and antibiotics used in commercial dairy products, there are plenty of good reasons for removing dairy from your diet. Many people rely on dairy as their main source of calcium, and it is a critical pregnancy nutrient to help your baby build strong bones and teeth, but there are many other food sources of calcium that can help you reach your goal of 1,000 milligrams per day. These include fish canned with bones (such as sardines and salmon), dark leafy greens, nuts and seeds, citrus fruits, dried fruits, and molasses. It all comes back to including an array of whole foods in your diet every day for maximum nutrient density!

ESSENTIAL

Most common pregnancy symptoms, including leg cramps, headaches, heartburn, constipation, hemorrhoids, swelling, bloating, fatigue, back pain, and trouble sleeping can be drastically improved with a healthy diet, proper hydration, regular exercise, low stress, and lots of shut-eye.

"Eating for Two"

You've surely heard the common myth that once you are carrying a baby you should start "eating for two." Since one of you starts out smaller than the size of a blueberry, you certainly don't need to eat twice as much. Actually, during pregnancy you only need a few hundred more calories per day than before you were pregnant. Your needs may vary slightly based on your pre-pregnancy weight or if you are carrying multiples, but this is really the equivalent of only a small meal or snack.

If you gain excess weight during pregnancy, you increase your risk of gestational diabetes, preeclampsia, and having a baby with high birth weight. On the other hand, if you don't gain enough weight during pregnancy, your baby may be born preterm or with a low birth weight. These all come with their own unique potential health concerns later in life, so always listen to your body's hunger cues and eat when you feel hungry, while keeping these caloric guidelines in mind. Remember: what you eat goes directly to your baby, so focus on food quality—meaning organic fruits and veggies and pastured meats—and variety so that you get the full range of important pregnancy nutrients.

CHAPTER 4

What to Expect During Each Trimester

Your pregnancy is measured in trimesters, starting from the first day of your last menstrual period, and lasting forty weeks. Each stage of pregnancy brings new changes, and with it excitement as your baby grows. Since you are following the Paleo diet and lifestyle, you are on your way to ensuring your baby receives the proper nutrients she needs to grow, and you're nourishing your body with healthful, whole foods. However, it is important to understand what happens during each trimester, and learn about the changes that are happening to your body and baby. This chapter breaks down the growth and changes month to month, so you'll know what to expect during the most important nine months of your life.

The First Trimester

Your first trimester of pregnancy ends at about twelve weeks, or three months after your last menstrual period. Your doctor may discuss your progress in weeks, which are measured from the first day of your last menstrual period—the day your doctor uses to calculate your due date and the baby's gestational age. (See Appendix E for a quick reference of estimated due dates.) Since it is usually impossible to pinpoint the exact date of ovulation and the date of conception, medical experts use your last menstrual period as the starting point for your next nine months. Basically, this means that the first week of your pregnancy is actually the week that you started your last period.

In terms of your lifestyle, it is important to take note that everything you eat, drink, and do will directly affect your baby. Experts don't exactly understand how the mother and baby divvy up the nutrients, but we do know that the baby lives on the nutrients from the mother's diet and the nutrients already stored in her bones and tissues. The baby's health and proper growth are directly related to the mother's diet before and during pregnancy—and by following the Paleo lifestyle, you and your baby will be getting the best nutrition possible. If you are not already taking a prenatal vitamin, now is a good time to start to ensure you are getting all of the nutrients that are essential to a healthy pregnancy, including folic acid, calcium, and iron. Good nutrition and a healthy lifestyle are essential throughout your entire pregnancy, though certain nutritional considerations may be more important at different stages along the way. In your first trimester, important nutritional considerations include folic acid intake, prevention of malnutrition, and dehydration.

What's Going On

Along with changes in your baby's development, you will experience changes in your own body. The embryo secretes a hormone called human chorionic gonadotropin (hCG), or the pregnancy hormone. This hormone triggers your first signs of pregnancy. In your first trimester, you may begin to experience nausea, vomiting, dizziness, headaches, a feeling of fullness or bloating, light cramping, constipation, poor appetite, frequent urination, and breast tenderness. You may need to go to the bathroom more often. This is because your growing uterus is pressing on your bladder and because hormones may be affecting your body's fluid balance.

Around week eight, your uterus grows from the size of your fist to about the size of a grapefruit, which can cause some mild cramping or pain in your lower abdomen or sides. Some of these problems will decrease as you continue with your pregnancy.

Moodiness and anxiety can surface and make you feel like you are on an emotional roller coaster. Feeling happy one day and crabby the next is completely normal, due partly to fluctuating and very high levels of hormones. For many women, this moodiness and anxiety continues throughout pregnancy. You may begin to notice changes in your figure by the end of your first trimester. Your breasts have become larger, and you may notice that your waistline is beginning to expand just a bit.

Average weight gain in the first trimester is anywhere from 1 to 5 pounds. You may gain more or you may even lose weight due to loss of appetite and morning sickness. Keep in mind that excessive weight gain during pregnancy can be a problem for both you and your baby. A normal weight gain during pregnancy, for women who begin at a normal weight, is 25 to 35 pounds. If your weight gain during the first trimester seems abnormal, speak with your doctor.

What's Happening with Baby?

Even though this is just the beginning, and your baby is tinier than you can probably imagine, it's a very big time for both of you! The development that occurs in these first few weeks is so rapid, and yet so essential to the healthy natural progression that will bring your baby from the bundle of cells he starts out as to the bundle of joy you'll soon deliver. You may feel pregnant, but you may not. You may start to show, but you may not. Regardless of what's happening on the outside, the miracles taking place in your body, each and every day, are nothing short of remarkable.

Your First Month (1 to 4 Weeks)

About two weeks after the first day of your last menstrual period, your ovary released an egg into the fallopian tube. Your actual pregnancy began when that egg was fertilized by a sperm cell.

Over the next week, the fertilized egg grows into a group of cells called a blastocyst. Once the blastocyst completes its journey down the fallopian tube, it implants in the uterus and divides into two parts. One half of the blastocyst attaches to the wall of the uterus and becomes the placenta while the other half develops into the embryo. This group of cells is already composed of different layers. The outer layer eventually becomes the nervous system, skin, and hair. The middle layer becomes bones, cartilage, muscles, circulatory system, kidneys, and sex organs. The inner layer becomes the respiratory and digestive organs.

The implantation of the egg into the uterus triggers the beginning of hormonal and physical changes. The amniotic sac, which cushions the fetus in the months ahead, begins to form. The early stages of the placenta and umbilical cord are visible and under rapid construction.

FACT

The placenta is the interface that provides all the nutrients the baby needs, including oxygen, and takes care of waste disposal. It also produces the hormones progesterone and estriol, which are produced to help maintain a healthy pregnancy. The placenta develops in the uterus just twelve days after conception.

During the first month of pregnancy, the embryo looks like a tadpole. The neural tube, which will become the brain and spinal cord, starts to come together. A very primitive face begins to form, with large dark circles where the eyes will be. The mouth, lower jaw, and throat also begin to develop. The baby's blood cells are taking shape, and circulation will soon begin. By the end of the first month, the embryo is about a quarter of an inch long and is smaller than a grain of rice.

Your Second Month (5 to 8 Weeks)

You may not look pregnant yet, but by the second month of your pregnancy, plenty is going on. Major body organs are beginning to develop, including the heart, brain, kidneys, liver, intestines, appendix, lungs, and body systems. The baby's facial features continue to develop. The baby's ears, fingers, toes, and eyes begin to form. Tiny buds that will become the baby's arms and legs are forming. The digestive tract and sensory organs are now beginning to develop.

During this time, bone starts to replace cartilage. The baby's heart starts its contractions, which will become distinct heartbeats within the next week. The eyelids form and grow—though sealed shut—and nostrils begin to form.

The neural tube will eventually connect the brain and spinal cord, and by about the fifth week it closes. Blood circulation becomes evident at this time. The placenta and amniotic sac continue to develop. By the end of the second month, the embryo has started to look more like a person than a tadpole. It measures about 1 inch long and weighs less than ⅛ ounce.

Your Third Month (9 to 12 Weeks)

During your third month of pregnancy, the embryo has developed into a fetus. The baby is active, even though you may not yet be able to feel the activity. All major organs, muscles, and nerves are formed. The mouth has twenty buds that will eventually become teeth. The irises of the eyes are now forming. The liver, intestines, brain, and lungs are now beginning to function on their own. At around week eleven, it is possible to hear the "swooshing" sound of the baby's heartbeat for the first time with a special instrument called a Doppler sound-wave stethoscope.

ESSENTIAL

A Doppler stethoscope uses ultrasound to listen to the heartbeat of the fetus. The device is sometimes called a Doptone. The Doppler may be routinely used during your prenatal visits.

Several of the baby's ribs are now visible, and tissue that will eventually form bones is developing around the baby's head, arms, and legs. By the end of your first trimester, or third month, your baby is fully formed. Your little one has arms, hands, fingers, feet, and toes. Fingers and toes are separate, and they now have soft nails. Your baby's reproductive organs are developing, and the circulatory and urinary systems are working. The liver is producing bile.

Throughout the remainder of your pregnancy, the baby's body organs will mature and the fetus will gain weight, become longer, and fully develop. By the end of your third month, your baby is about four inches in length and weighs about 1 ounce. The most critical point of formation of the organs is finished, and your chance of miscarriage at this point drops considerably.

The Second Trimester

In your second trimester of pregnancy, you will begin to gain more of your pregnancy weight. You should experience a steady weight gain of about 1 pound per week in your second trimester, although the rate of weight gain differs from woman to woman. Even though your body may be changing, keep in mind that proper weight gain is a good thing in pregnancy because it means your baby is growing normally. If you are struggling with your changing figure, don't beat yourself up about feeling a little unhappy. It is very normal, and you should give yourself permission to experience both the joys and frustrations of watching your body change in so many ways.

What's Going On

The changes in the second trimester can be quite dramatic. You might wake up one morning and feel like a cloud has been lifted. You may not even feel very pregnant in the classic sense of nausea and grouchiness. Where you may have felt exhausted, cranky, mentally foggy, and an overall sense of being uncomfortable, the second trimester will probably be your turnaround point where you get to feel like yourself again. Not only will you be feeling better accustomed to being pregnant, but you may get the sense that your body is, too.

If you weren't showing much in your first trimester and felt like wearing a sign that read, "I'm pregnant!" to let people in on your excitement, your second trimester will take care of your hidden condition by being the time when you "pop" your baby belly that will let everyone know you're expecting. With your expanding belly, you get to explore the whole new world of maternity wear that will help you feel comfortable and stylish. With more energy, less discomfort, a new wardrobe, and a proud baby bump, what's not to feel great about? Add to all of the second-trimester greatness the fact that you get to feel your baby move for the first time, and you may just feel like it can't get any better!

Be sure to take advantage of this pregnancy period. Use the time to get out and enjoy life. Take more walks; spend more time doing things you enjoy. Simply enjoy the pregnancy.

What's Happening with Baby?

By your second trimester, your baby is well developed. This stage of the pregnancy can be very exciting because you may start to feel your baby move at about eighteen to twenty-two weeks. If this is not your first pregnancy, you may even be able to feel movement earlier, at sixteen to eighteen weeks. Your baby looks like a small person now and is continuing to develop every week during this period.

Your Fourth Month (13 to 16 Weeks)

By your fourth month of pregnancy, your baby's fingers and toes are well defined. Eyelids, eyebrows, and nails are formed. Hair is starting to grow on top of the baby's head, and facial features are more prominent. The teeth and bones are becoming harder. The baby is moving her arms and legs and can even suck her thumb, yawn, and stretch. The baby is starting to now respond to outside stimuli. The nervous system is beginning to function, and the reproductive organs and genitalia are now fully developed. At this point your doctor may be able tell through an ultrasound if you are having a boy or a girl. The baby's heartbeat is now undeniably audible through an instrument called a Doppler. By the end of your fourth month, the baby is about six inches long and weighs somewhere around 4 ounces.

Your Fifth Month (17 to 20 Weeks)

During your fifth month of pregnancy, hair on the head, eyebrows, and eyelashes is filling in. A soft, fine hair, called lanugo, covers the baby's body. Meant to protect the baby, lanugo is usually shed by the end of the baby's first week of life. Fat is beginning to form on the baby's body to help him stay warm and to aid in metabolism. The lungs, circulatory, and urinary systems are now in working condition. At this point, the retinas in the eyes are sensitive to light. The baby's skin is developing and appears transparent. Your baby can hear sounds such as your voice and heartbeat as well as sounds outside of your body. During this month, you may begin to feel the baby move as his muscles begin to develop. As the baby continues to develop, you will notice more movement. By the end of the fifth month, the baby is about ten inches long and weighs anywhere from 8 ounces to 1 pound.

FACT

At this point, you should start sleeping on your side because the circulation is best for mom and baby that way. By the time you get to your fourth or fifth month, lying on your stomach or your back can put extra pressure on your growing uterus and may decrease circulation to the baby.

Your Sixth Month (21 to 25 Weeks)

During your sixth month, the baby is continuing to gain fat to keep his body warm. His growth rate is slowing down, but bodily systems such as digestion are continuing to mature. Buds for the permanent teeth are beginning to form, and the baby's muscles are getting stronger. The baby is very active and will respond to sounds and movement. The baby's body is becoming better proportioned. It is beginning to produce white blood cells that will help the baby fight infection and disease. You may begin to tell when the baby has hiccups by the jerking motions you feel. The baby's skin is more opaque than transparent and is wrinkled as the baby grows into it. The heartbeat at this point can be heard more easily through a stethoscope, depending on the baby's position. By the end of the sixth month, your baby measures approximately twelve inches in length and somewhere around 2 pounds.

What Your Body Needs

As with your entire pregnancy, good nutrition and proper weight gain are essential during your second trimester. During this period, most women begin to experience decreased symptoms of morning sickness (though some may get morning sickness throughout pregnancy). It's a good thing these symptoms decrease for most because you need to continue to boost your calorie intake. The nutritional concerns in this stage of pregnancy come from the digestive troubles that most women begin to experience.

As your pregnancy progresses into the second trimester, your baby continues to grow, which causes your stomach to work a little slower. Some women may experience digestive problems as they enter the second trimester, including gas, indigestion, and heartburn. Constipation can become a problem during the second trimester and continue until the end of your pregnancy. It is important to deal with these discomforts so that they don't interfere with your efforts to eat a healthy Paleo diet and don't turn into more complex complications.

The Third Trimester

By your last trimester, you will have put on much of your pregnancy weight as your baby fully grows and develops. You should still be gaining weight at a rate of about 1 pound per week. You will probably begin to feel some pain in the ribs as your baby grows and pushes upward on your rib cage. The pressure may also give you some indigestion and heartburn. You may begin to see stretch marks as your uterus expands. Your balance and mobility will also change as you get bigger. Throughout your last trimester, as your baby continues to grow, you will begin to experience some discomforts such as leg cramps, mild swelling of the feet and ankles, constipation, difficulty with sleep, shortness of breath, lower abdominal pain, backaches, and Braxton Hicks contractions. You may feel a more frequent urge to urinate again as you did in the first trimester.

All women "carry" differently. Some will carry the baby higher or lower, bigger or smaller, wider or more compact. All these depend on the size and position of your little one, your body type, and how much body weight you have gained.

By your ninth month, your weight gain should be somewhere around 24 to 29 pounds. It may get more uncomfortable to sleep and move around, and it is normal to become moody and irritable. As you near the end, you may notice alternating feelings of fatigue and bursts of energy.

FACT

Around your twenty-eighth to thirtieth week of pregnancy, or even as early as twenty weeks, you may experience episodes in which your belly tightens, becomes firm, and then relaxes. This feeling, which is very normal, comes from contractions of the uterine muscles called Braxton Hicks contractions. They are a type of warmup or practice for the uterus for labor. Braxton Hicks contractions usually occur no more than four to six times per hour in your ninth month. If you can't tell the difference between Braxton Hicks contractions and true labor contractions, ask your doctor.

It is a good time to think ahead and prepare for your return from the hospital . . . with a newborn! Use those energy bursts to start stocking your freezer with foods you can easily pop in your oven or microwave. Cook casseroles, chili, soups, and other dishes that can be frozen and prepared later when you are too busy to worry about cooking.

What's Going On

The final stretch of the pregnancy journey has finally begun. As you've learned to adapt to the physical and mental changes throughout pregnancy, the third trimester is no different. As you get closer to your due date, you may find that fatigue and insomnia once again begin to plague you. These complaints are very common for pregnant women in their third trimester due to the great changes that are taking place in their minds and bodies as they prepare for the birth of their baby. While annoying, none of these troubles are life-threatening and most of these temporary discomforts can be resolved naturally.

FACT

During the course of your pregnancy, your body will produce approximately 50 percent more blood and body fluids to meet the needs of your developing baby. The accumulation of these extra fluids accounts for almost 25 percent of a woman's weight gain during pregnancy.

What's Happening with Baby?

During your last trimester, your baby continues to grow larger, and his body organs continue to mature. Your baby is completing his development for his introduction to the world. With your baby growing and getting heavier, the last three months can get a bit uncomfortable—just keep thinking about the end result!

Your Seventh Month (26 to 30 Weeks)

Your baby will really start squirming around between the twenty-seventh and thirty-second weeks. Starting with your seventh month, the baby's lungs continue to develop, but they are not yet fully mature. To practice waking up Mom and Dad at all hours of the night, the baby begins to develop patterns of waking and sleeping. The baby's hands are active, and fingernails are growing. Muscle coordination is getting much better. The baby can now suck his thumb and can even cry. By week twenty-eight, the baby's eyelids are opening. The lungs are developed enough that if the baby were born prematurely, he would have a good chance at survival but would need to stay in a neonatal intensive care unit (NICU). As your seventh month progresses and the baby grows larger, he experiences a harder time moving around in the uterus due to space constraints. However, he still seems to find the room to do some kicking and stretching. The baby gains more fat on his body to help control his own temperature.

By the end of this month, the eyebrows and eyelashes are filled in and any hair the baby has on his head is becoming thicker. The head is now proportioned to the rest of the body. The baby's hearing is fully developed, and he can respond to stimuli such as pain, light, and sounds. Toward the end of this month amniotic fluid begins to diminish. Your baby now measures about seventeen inches from head to toe and weighs about 2 to 4 pounds.

ALERT

Around the seventh month of your pregnancy, it is normal for your blood pressure to increase slightly. However, you should contact your doctor if you experience severe headaches, blurred vision, or severe swelling in your hands, feet, and/or ankles. These specific symptoms could signal the beginning of a condition called preeclampsia, which is pregnancy-induced hypertension, or high blood pressure.

Your Eighth Month (31 to 34 Weeks)

Starting with your eighth month, the baby is becoming too big to move easily inside the uterus. It may seem that the baby is moving less. The baby is developing more fat beneath his thin layer of skin, and he's starting to practice opening his eyes. Most of his internal systems and organs are now well developed except the lungs, which are not quite yet fully matured. The baby's brain continues to develop at a rapid pace. These weeks mark a ton of growth for the baby. During the last seven weeks, the baby gains more than half his birth weight. As the baby becomes larger, he begins to run out of room and takes the fetal position by curling up. By the end of the eighth month, the baby begins to move into a head-down position, although that may not be his final position at birth. Your baby now measures around 19.8 inches from head to toe and weighs about 5 pounds.

Your Ninth Month (35 to 40 Weeks)

By nine months, your baby's lungs are almost fully developed. He still doesn't have quite enough fat under the skin to keep himself warm outside of the womb, but he is working on it. By the ninth month, the baby begins to drop lower into your abdomen, usually with the head in a downward position. The brain has been rapidly developing, and the baby's reflexes are coordinated so he can blink his eyes, turn his head, grasp firmly with his hands, and respond to stimuli. Every day, the baby is taking on a rounder shape, developing pinker skin, and losing his wrinkled appearance. The baby is beginning to get antibodies from you that will help protect him from illness.

In this last month, the growth of your baby tends to slow down, yet he is still collecting fat under his skin and, therefore, putting on more weight. The toenails have grown to the tips of the toes, as have the fingernails, which have grown to the tips of the fingers. The baby's arm and leg muscles are stronger, and he is beginning to practice breathing and working out his lungs. By the end of the ninth month, your baby will drop farther into your pelvis, hopefully with head aimed downward to the birth canal, to prepare for delivery. The drop of the baby will help you breathe a little easier. Your baby's length at birth is about 18 to 20 inches on average, and he weighs about 7.5 pounds. Length and weight vary greatly from baby to baby.

CHAPTER 5

Pregnancy and Fitness

Regular exercise during pregnancy goes hand in hand with proper nutrition. There was a time when pregnant women were advised to put their feet up and avoid exercise, but that is no longer the case. The ACOG currently recommends at least thirty minutes of physical activity on most days. If you are already exercising regularly, there is no reason to stop now, and if you do not currently have an exercise routine, now is a great time to start. With a few modifications and the go-ahead from your health care provider, exercise should definitely be a part of your pregnancy. Not only will exercise help you reduce your risk of many pregnancy complications, find relief from common pregnancy symptoms, and bounce back more quickly from labor and delivery, but it can also inspire you to embrace your changing body and connect with your baby.

Exercise Benefits for Mom and Baby

Exercise during pregnancy is important for you and your baby. Exercise increases circulation, which helps to deliver nutrients to your baby via the placenta and to clear toxins from your body. It also builds muscle tone and fitness of the uterus, making you better prepared to handle pregnancy and childbirth. The perks of regular physical activity during pregnancy also include:

- Fewer aches and pains
- Reduced swelling and discomfort
- Healthy digestion
- Improved sleep quality
- Prevention of excess weight gain
- Increased energy and stamina
- Fewer mood swings
- Reduced risk of diabetes and preeclampsia
- Shorter and easier labor
- Faster recovery from delivery

The benefits extend to your baby, as well. Babies born to mothers who exercise regularly during pregnancy are more likely to be born at a healthy birth weight, which reduces the risk of birth injuries and interventions such as C-section or forceps delivery that are often necessary for high birth weight babies. A 2013 study in *Early Human Development* actually showed that regular exercise improves a baby's cardiovascular health in utero and into childhood.

FACT

In the 2013 *Early Human Development* study, babies born to mothers who exercised for at least thirty minutes, three times per week had lower heart rates and increased heart rate variability in utero and in infancy than those whose mothers did not exercise during pregnancy. For healthy individuals, having a lower heart rate means your heart doesn't have to work as hard because it is delivering more oxygen through your blood with each beat.

While still inconclusive, there are recent human studies that suggest babies born to moms who exercise during pregnancy have more mature brains. In a presentation at the 2013 Society for Neurosicence annual meeting, researchers found that babies born to mothers who exercised at least 20 minutes per day three times per week were able to recognize new sounds with less effort than babies born to mothers who did not exercise during pregnancy. Researchers are continuing to monitor these babies to see if the findings hold true into childhood. As you can see, regular exercise during pregnancy is just what the doctor ordered, as long as you know which exercises to enjoy and which ones to avoid.

Changing Your Athletic Performance

This is not the time to beat your previous half-marathon time or set a personal record for your deadlift. Right now, exercise is all about maintaining your current fitness level and preparing your body for pregnancy, labor, delivery, and postpartum recovery. If you are having a normal, healthy pregnancy, you should be able to continue with your current exercise regimen with a few modifications. If you were not exercising prior to getting pregnant, now is a great time to start.

Because every pregnancy is different, speak with your health care provider before starting an exercise program or continuing with your current routine to discuss any specific sports or movements to avoid, potential risks to you and your baby, and any modifications that need to be made. You should also talk with any athletic coaches or fitness instructors you are working with, even if you haven't yet spilled the beans to friends and family that you are pregnant. It is important that they know you are pregnant so they can offer modification techniques and help you avoid any unsafe movements. Take plenty of rest breaks, remember to fuel up before and after working out, and drink lots of water.

Best Pregnancy Activities

If you are just starting an exercise routine, there are certain guidelines to keep in mind. You want to start slow and focus on gradually increasing time, intensity, and frequency to work up to at least the recommended thirty minutes, but only at a level that feels comfortable for you. Walking is a great place to start, but there are plenty of exercises that are safe to begin even after you find out you are pregnant. Some of the best activities for moms-to-be include:

- **Running:** If you were an avid runner pre-pregnancy, you should be able to continue unless it becomes too uncomfortable. You may find that you tire out more quickly, so take walking breaks as needed. And don't be surprised if you need a few extra bathroom breaks, too, because of hormone changes and the extra pressure your growing uterus is putting on your bladder.

- **Swimming and water aerobics:** Swimming is an excellent full-body exercise with both cardiovascular and muscle-strengthening benefits. If you are not a fan of lap swimming, sign up for a water aerobics class at your local gym. You'll perform many of the same movements that you would in a typical aerobics class, but without the added impact on your joints.

- **Low-impact aerobics:** With just a quick search, you can find countless DVDs and online aerobics workouts geared toward pregnant women to keep your heart in top shape. If you are a beginner or just prefer a group environment, take a class at your local gym with a reputable, qualified instructor; just be sure to let her know you are pregnant.

- **Stationary bike:** Some pregnant women may feel comfortable riding their bike through most of their pregnancy, but if you are accident-prone or feeling the effects of your changing center of gravity, you may prefer a stationary bike. Cycling provides a good aerobic workout and strengthens your legs. Most gyms have a selection to choose from so you can cycle at your own pace, or you can hit up a spin class.

- **Weight training:** Weight training increases all-over muscle tone and strength to help your body better handle pregnancy and prepare for delivery. If you are new to weight training, always work with a certified trainer either one-on-one or in a class setting at your gym. If you are used to strength training, focus on maintaining your current level of fitness and proper form. Certain lifts can put a lot of stress on your lower back, and you may have more difficulty keeping your balance, so decrease weight as needed and ask your trainer for modifications.

- **Prenatal Pilates:** Pilates is wonderful during pregnancy because it strengthens and tones your core and pelvic floor muscles. Just as with other types of pregnancy exercise, you can find at-home or in-class options, and even private Pilates instructors. You just have to know your experience level and how much personalized instruction you need.

- **Prenatal yoga:** Not only is prenatal yoga a great method to strengthen your whole body, including your core, it also gives you a gentle all-over stretch and teaches you useful relaxation techniques, such as deep breathing, that can even be used during labor. If you already partici-pate in a yoga practice, let the instructor know as soon as you find out you are pregnant so he can offer modifications. If you prefer to practice in the privacy of your own living room, search specifically for prenatal yoga videos.

QUESTION

Where do I find prenatal fitness classes?
There are tons of resources for finding all types of prenatal fitness classes and breaking a sweat with other moms-to-be. Check with the hospital or birthing center where you plan to deliver, your health care provider or doula, your birth education instructor, a local baby store, the YMCA, or other local gyms. You can even take your search online to sites like Meetup.com to find other fitness-minded moms in your area.

First Trimester

In the first trimester, extreme fatigue and nausea may push exercise to the bottom of your list. If your energy tank is running on empty, try not to beat yourself up over it and just do what you can, even if it is only a short walk. Even cleaning the house and folding the laundry might feel like a workout! If you can't drag yourself out of bed and you do miss a workout, don't worry. When you feel up to a workout, not many modifications will be necessary in the first trimester because your body usually doesn't change too much in those first few months. Anything you were doing prior to getting pregnant, you should be able to continue with. Just take breaks as needed, drink plenty of water, and do what feels right for you.

Second Trimester

For most women, energy levels come bouncing back by the second trimester and you may see an increase in your physical performance from the first trimester. This is also the time, though, when your body begins to change and grow more rapidly; therefore, certain exercise modifications become necessary. While you should still be able to continue with your normal routine, don't do anything that feels uncomfortable to you. There are a few changes you will want to be aware of now and for the remainder of your pregnancy:

- **Your center of gravity shifts:** As your body grows and changes during pregnancy, your center of gravity tends to shift upward. This can leave you feeling a bit wobbly and more likely to lose your balance while working out. Move slowly and use extra caution when performing movements where you could easily lose your footing, such as lunges, running, or one-legged yoga postures. This is especially true once your belly grows large enough that you can no longer see your feet. Core strengthening exercises can also help counteract these changes.
- **Lying flat on your back is hazardous:** When you lie down, your growing uterus can put pressure on the vena cava, a major vein that delivers blood to the heart. This can cause you to feel faint and dizzy, which is why doctors will usually advise that you refrain from exercises like sit-ups and crunches after the fourth month of pregnancy. Instead, use a stability ball for support in an inclined position, and focus on other types of core-strengthening exercises such as planks or push-ups.
- **Standing in place is also hazardous:** Similar to lying flat on your back, standing motionless for too long can reduce blood flow and leave you feeling woozy. Keep this in mind if you participate in yoga, tai chi, or Pilates.
- **Your body is extra limber:** You have the hormone relaxin to thank for those extra-loose limbs and joints, especially in your hips, pelvis, and lower back. This allows your muscles to stretch during delivery, but it can influence your workouts, too. But just because you can bend and stretch deeper than you're used to doesn't mean you should. Be careful not to overstretch when doing squats, lunges, and similar movements.
- **Now-risky activities should be avoided:** Certain activities, such as horseback riding, mounting climbing, and soccer, have a higher risk of injury

than others. Any type of exercise or sport with a high risk for falling or abdominal trauma could pose a hazard to you and your baby.

QUESTION

What is diastasis recti?
Diastasis recti is a separation of the left and right sides of the abdominal muscles and can occur during pregnancy because of increased tension on the abdominal wall. Diastasis recti can't always be avoided, but you run a greater risk if you are carrying multiples, have had previous pregnancies, or if you have poor abdominal muscle tone. It occurs most often in the second and third trimesters and can affect the strength of your abdominal muscles even after birth. Your provider can give you a confirmed diagnosis and instruct you on movements to avoid, but if you notice a bulge in the middle of your belly or feel a gap in your abdominal muscles when you lie down, you may have diastasis recti.

Third Trimester

The third trimester often brings its own set of challenges. Many women experience a lot of hip and back pain, thanks again to the relaxin hormone. You may also have swelling in your feet and ankles or shortness of breath, and some of that first-trimester fatigue may return. Again, do whatever activities you can. Because physical activity prepares your body for labor, try to make it a part of your daily routine. If you are experiencing any aches and pains and can't exercise as you normally do, try swimming or water aerobics. Swimming is great for moving your baby into the right position for labor; it relieves swelling and the strain on your joints, and it just makes you feel good by letting you be weightless for a while. The calming movement of the water is also a great stress reliever. If you are in so much pain you can barely walk from the couch to the refrigerator for a snack, talk with your practitioner. She can give you focused stretches and strengthening exercises or refer you to a chiropractor or physical therapist.

There are specific exercises you can focus on during the third trimester to get your body in tip-top shape for labor and delivery. Strengthening your pelvic floor by doing Kegel exercises minimizes the stress put on these muscles during pregnancy and increases circulation to your vaginal area, which speeds healing after birth and helps your pelvic floor return to its pre-pregnancy state. You'll need to continue with these exercises after you give birth to continue to strengthen these muscles. You can also do pelvic tilts to strengthen your core and ease back pain during pregnancy and labor. Search YouTube (*www.youtube.com*) for instructional videos on how to perform these exercises.

Safety Considerations for Mom and Baby

Regular exercise during pregnancy is a wonderful way to care for yourself and your baby. You've already discovered the long list of benefits, but there are safety considerations to keep in mind as well. First and foremost, it is essential that you listen to your body. Rest when you need to, drink plenty of water, and even eat a small snack if you feel hungry five minutes into your workout. If anything feels uncomfortable, painful, or "just not right," honor what your body is telling you and stop.

ESSENTIAL

Finding out you're pregnant is the perfect excuse to go shopping for some new workout gear. Your growing breasts need a supportive (and probably larger) sports bra, your feet may swell enough that you need to go up a size in your running shoes, and many women choose to invest in a pregnancy belt to support their belly and lower back during exercise. Pick up a few cute maternity workout tops while you're at it!

As mentioned earlier, there are a few high-risk activities you want to avoid during pregnancy, especially sports and exercises that pose a danger of falling or of abdominal injury. If you participate in any of these activities, talk with your health care provider to discuss safety precautions and/or alternatives. These include, but are not limited to:

- Contact sports (basketball, soccer, hockey, etc.)
- Horseback riding
- Mountain biking
- Racquet sports

- Scuba diving
- Skiing (water or downhill snow)
- Snowboarding

Even if your practitioner gives you the "a-okay" on your workout plan, your body may tell you otherwise. If you experience the following warning signs, stop exercising immediately. If they don't resolve quickly on their own after rest, rehydration, and a small snack, then contact your health care provider.

- Blurred vision
- Calf pain or swelling
- Chest pain
- Contractions
- Decreased fetal movement
- Dizziness
- Headache
- Muscle weakness
- Nausea
- Overheating
- Rapid heartbeat
- Shortness of breath
- Vaginal bleeding/leakage

While regular exercise is often advised to prevent and manage pregnancy conditions such as gestational diabetes, there are certain conditions that may force you to limit or avoid physical activity. Depending on your unique situation, there are some low-impact movements and activities like walking that may still be safe for you. The ACOG currently recommends avoiding aerobic exercise if you suffer from any of the following:

- Hypertension (diagnosed pre-pregnancy or due to preeclampsia)
- Fetal growth restriction (below the 10th percentile for gestational age)
- Hyperthyroidism
- Incompetent cervix (when the cervix begins to open too early during pregnancy, before the baby is fully developed)
- Lung disease (e.g., asthma, severe bronchitis)

- Persistent bleeding
- Placenta previa (when the placenta covers all or part of the opening to the cervix)
- Premature labor
- Ruptured membranes
- Seizure disorder
- Severe anemia

If you have a history with any of these health issues or develop them during pregnancy, talk with your provider. She can suggest the types and amount of exercise that are safe for you. It may be difficult to rest when you are used to being active, but remember that this is a temporary and necessary restriction, for your safety and the safety of your baby.

Pre-Workout Nutrition

Fueling up before a workout is always a good idea, but even more so when you are pregnant. Your body is already using extra energy and nutrients even when you are at rest, so you need to make sure you are taking in extra food to make up for the calories you'll burn during exercise. Eat a meal or snack about sixty minutes before your workout so your body has time to digest the food. Even if you are the type of person who likes to wake up and get your workout out of the way, give yourself enough time to eat a small snack before getting started. You will want to include complex carbohydrates and lean protein in your pre-workout meal. Carbohydrates are your body's preferred fuel of choice for more intense workouts, such as cycling, running, swimming, and aerobics. They are also easily digested, so your body won't be bogged down trying to digest your food and you'll have more energy for your workout. Protein is satiating, so you won't feel hungry while you work out, and it will help with post-workout recovery and muscle repair. Small amounts of fats are fine, too, but too much fat before a workout can leave you feeling sluggish. These pre-workout meal and snack ideas offer everything you need to feel strong and energized throughout your workout:

- Banana and almond butter
- Banana Berry Smoothie (see Chapter 15)

- Cinnamon Baked Sweet Potato (see Chapter 14)
- Dried apricots and beef jerky
- Garden Veggie Omelet (see Chapter 7)
- Grapes, baby carrots, and organic deli turkey meat
- Paleo Trail Mix Bars (see Chapter 17) and an apple
- Salmon and Citrus Salad (see Chapter 13)

You may be used to powering through a workout without much to drink, but pregnancy changes the rules of the game. You need to drink plenty of water to replace water lost through sweat and to keep from overheating and dehydrating. On top of the recommended eight (8-ounce) glasses of water per day, drink an 8-ounce glass of water with your pre-workout meal. Add in another 8 ounces for every thirty minutes of exercise, more if you are exercising in hot and humid conditions. Don't wait until you are thirsty to drink; keep your water bottle handy and sip throughout your workout. If you stop sweating, experience cramping, or feel faint or dizzy, stop working out immediately and rehydrate.

Post-Workout Nutrition

Post-workout is all about recovery. The focus should be on mostly protein with some carbohydrates thrown in as well. A small amount of healthy fat is okay here, too. Carbohydrates replenish your body's glycogen stores, which become depleted during exercise. Protein facilitates this process and also stimulates muscle growth and repair. When you perform weight-bearing exercise, such as running or weight-lifting, it creates tiny tears in your muscles. Protein repairs those tears and rebuilds your muscles, making you stronger with every workout. Good choices include:

- Banana Pancakes topped with walnuts (see Chapter 7)
- California Salad (see Chapter 13)
- Cinnamon Baked Sweet Potato (see Chapter 14)
- Baked Chicken and Peppers (see Chapter 10)
- Lettuce-Wrapped Bison Burgers (see Chapter 9)
- Paleo BLT (see Chapter 17)
- Two hard-boiled eggs, sugar snap peas, and an orange

It's not just what you eat, but also *when* you eat that is important. For maximum recovery and muscle-building benefits, eat your post-workout meal within thirty to sixty minutes of completing your workout. Your body begins the repair process as soon as you stop exercising, so consuming your post-workout meal during this window will speed recovery and lessen fatigue and muscle soreness. Don't forget to down another 8 ounces of water with your recovery meal to make up for any fluid lost during your workout. You may need even more on hot and humid days. Eating soup or broth after a workout can also help your body to rehydrate.

CHAPTER 6

The Postpartum Paleo Body

If you thought giving birth was the end of crazy hormones and extreme body changes, you will soon learn that the postpartum period brings its own set of transformations and challenges. Some of these developments are miraculous, such as the fact that your body can actually create food for your baby, and some can be frustrating, like finding time to brush your teeth and take a shower. Nutrition, physical activity, and rest are just as important now as they were during pregnancy, but for different reasons. Read on to learn all about how to navigate this new way of life with your little one and soak up every precious moment.

Breastfeeding

You'll begin to notice changes in your breasts during pregnancy as your body prepares for milk production. They tend to grow a size or two, and they may leak colostrum before you even give birth. Colostrum is the first milk that your breasts produce, and while there may not be much of it, it actually contains high levels of antibodies and immunoglobulins that begin to build healthy bacteria in your baby's gut and protect her from infection. Over the next few days to a week, colostrum production will gradually transition as your milk comes in. Most women are very much aware of this transition because their breasts will become engorged with milk and may even feel sore. Allowing your baby to nurse often will relieve the swelling and pressure. Usually your body will get more in tune with your baby's nursing schedule as time passes, and your body will learn how much milk to produce and when. Unlike cow or sheep's dairy, human milk perfectly matches the nutritional needs of your baby and actually adapts over time as your baby grows and changes. It contains the ideal balance of protein, fat, and carbohydrates, plus vitamins and minerals, digestive enzymes, and the same immunological benefits as colostrum.

FACT

Did you know that more than half of the calories in breast milk come from fats? Some of these fats are made in the body, while others are passed through breast milk from the dietary fat you consume. Breast milk also contains the enzyme lipase to help your baby digest and absorb this fat.

Benefits of Breastfeeding

The benefits of breastfeeding range from antibacterial, antimicrobial, and antiviral properties to lowered risk of certain diseases later in life. These beneficial properties increase in relation to how long you breastfeed. And breastfeeding doesn't only benefit your baby; there are perks for mom, too. Here is a rundown of some of the many benefits of breastfeeding for both mom and baby according to La Leche League International, a worldwide organization dedicated to providing information and support to breastfeeding mothers:

- Strengthens your baby's immune system and promotes healthy gut bacteria, possibly lifelong
- Decreases your baby's risk of developing certain food allergies
- Is an exact nutritional match to your baby's needs
- Reduces your baby's risk of being overweight later in life
- Is free and readily available
- If done for at least a month, gives you a lower risk of heart disease, high blood pressure, diabetes, high cholesterol, and stroke
- Reduces your risk of breast and ovarian cancer
- Provides comfort and bonding time with your baby
- Stimulates contractions in the uterus to prevent postpartum hemorrhage and speed the return of the uterus to its pre-pregnancy size
- Delays return of menstruation, thus acting as a natural form of birth control
- Burns calories and can help you return to your pre-pregnancy weight sooner

How a Paleo Diet Supports Breastfeeding

A healthy Paleo diet goes hand in hand with a healthy breast milk supply. In order for your body to produce the highest quality milk, you need to feed it the highest quality foods. Because milk production requires energy, you also need to make sure you are eating and drinking enough to support your milk supply. If you aren't drinking enough water, your milk supply can take a hit, so try to stick with the eight (8-ounce) cups per day that you were drinking during pregnancy. Breastfeeding mothers need about an extra 500 calories per day from healthy whole foods—not much more than the extra calories needed during pregnancy—but follow your hunger cues and do not deprive yourself if you feel hungry. Now is not the time to focus on getting back into your skinny jeans (although breastfeeding does often help that happen faster). Instead, remember that you need to nourish your own body in order to nourish your baby. Continue to include a variety of fresh fruits and vegetables, meat, nuts, and seafood to get all of the protein, fat, and carbohydrates you need. Here's why:

- **Protein:** At 71 grams per day, the RDA for protein for lactating women is almost twice as high as for non-pregnant, non-lactating women. Proteins are literally the building blocks of every type of cell and tissue in your body, from organs and muscles to hair and nails. The protein content of your breast milk is related to your dietary protein intake, so you need to consume enough to support your baby's growing body.
- **Fat:** The fat and cholesterol content of breast milk is highest during infancy because babies need fats to support growth and brain and nervous system development. Infancy is a time of rapid growth, and your dietary fat intake influences the fat content of your milk. Cholesterol is an important component in the protective covering of your baby's cell membranes. Because babies need fat from saturated and unsaturated sources to get all of the essential fatty acids, fill up on an assortment of fatty fish, red meat, pork, eggs, nuts and seeds (and their oils), avocados, and coconut.
- **Carbohydrates:** Carbohydrates provide fuel for both your body and your baby's. Your body is burning through energy to make milk, so it is important that you get lots of fresh fruits and vegetables to protect your milk supply.

ESSENTIAL

Coconut oil is packed with healthy fats, but it is famous for its many other uses as well. Coconut oil is very moisturizing and has antimicrobial and antifungal properties. It can be used to relieve dry, cracked nipples, and it can be used to help treat yeast that causes thrush in babies and moms.

Vitamin and Mineral Needs During Lactation

Your health care provider may advise you to continue taking your prenatal vitamin while you are breastfeeding to make sure you continue to meet the RDAs and support your baby's growth and development. The RDAs during lactation are as follows.

RECOMMENDED DIETARY ALLOWANCES DURING LACTATION	
Calcium	1,300 mg (milligrams)
Choline	550 mg
Copper	1,300 mcg (micrograms)
DHA	1,300 mg
Folate	500 mcg
Iodine	290 mcg
Iron	10 mg
Magnesium	310–360 mg
Niacin	17 mg
Riboflavin	1.6 mg
Selenium	70 mcg
Thiamin	1.4 mg
Vitamin A	1,200 mcg
Vitamin B$_6$	2.0 mg
Vitamin B$_{12}$	2.8 mcg
Vitamin C	120 mg
Vitamin D	600 IU (International Units)
Vitamin E	19 mg
Vitamin K	90 mcg
Zinc	13 mg

Source: Food and Nutrition Board, Institute of Medicine, National Academies

As you can see, the RDAs for lactation are similar to RDAs during pregnancy, with a few key differences. Calcium recommendations increase because, according to a 2005 study in the *Journal of Perinatal Education*, a mother can transfer as much as 1,000 milligrams per day to her baby through breast milk. Without adequate calcium intake, your own body's calcium stores can quickly diminish, leaving you at risk for osteoporosis later in life. Luckily, research also shows that your bones will remineralize after breastfeeding and bone density will increase. Vitamin A and vitamin C needs are also higher than pregnancy levels because these vitamins are secreted in high amounts through milk. It is also important that you continue to include omega-3 fatty acids by consuming fish and dark leafy greens to support your baby's brain, immune, and nervous system development. Omega-3s help your body to absorb the fat-soluble vitamins, A, D, E, and K, too. Because most infants do not receive enough regular sun exposure to meet their vitamin D requirements, the CDC now recommends that women who exclusively breastfeed give their baby a supplement of 400 IU per day of vitamin D to ensure they are getting enough of this bone-strengthening nutrient.

Making Time for Good Nutrition

You know what you should be eating, but how are you supposed to make time to feed yourself a healthy diet when you are spending all day (and night) feeding and caring for your baby? Here are a few tips for getting in those extra calories and nutrients while juggling life with a newborn:

- **Keep a nursing caddy:** Fill a small box or basket with everything you need to have handy for breastfeeding, such as hand lotion and a burp cloth, and include healthy snacks and a water bottle. Stock the caddy with apples, oranges, nuts, dried fruits, and Paleo Trail Mix Bars (see Chapter 17) and you can eat when your baby does. Get a caddy that is easily portable so you can move it around the house or take it on the go.
- **Meal planning:** By taking a little time (probably while your baby is snoozing) to plan your meals for the week, you can ensure you've got food in the house for all of your meals and snacks. A trip to the grocery store takes on a whole new meaning when you have an infant in tow, so you want to be able to get everything you need in one trip and have it at home and ready to go. Refer to the meal plans in Appendix A for some ideas to get you started.
- **Keep a water bottle by your side:** All day and all night, keep your water bottle close by and refill it often. Most breastfeeding moms are quite thirsty, especially in the early days, so you may not need much reminding, but if it helps you to remember, try to drink some water every time your baby eats.
- **Grab-and-go foods:** You don't want to spend all your free time cooking when you could be spending it with your snuggly newborn, so keep plenty of easy grab-and-go foods around, such as hard-boiled eggs,

veggie sticks, grapes, berries, jerky, and organic deli meat or cold lefto-ver meats.

QUESTION

Where can I find support if I am having difficulty breastfeeding? Breastfeeding doesn't always come easy. Whether your baby has trou-ble latching, you are experiencing pain and discomfort, or you just need tips on how to comfortably hold your baby, help is a phone call away. Contact your health care provider, local hospital, or baby store and they can refer you to a professionally trained and highly experi-enced International Board Certified Lactation Consultant (IBCLC). A doula can also offer support, or you can connect with other breast-feeding moms through local support groups or a nearby chapter of La Leche League (*www.llli.org*).

Alternatives to Breastfeeding

Even if you have a grand plan to breastfeed your baby, your body (or your baby) might have other plans. Sometimes you can't breastfeed because of low milk supply, allergies, or certain illnesses or medications—or your baby may flat-out refuse to nurse. You might have personal reasons for choosing not to breastfeed, and that is perfectly okay. As a mother, you will have to make decisions for your baby every day, and you have to do what works best for you. Your happiness and stress levels are directly related to your over-all health, so if you've considered the pros and cons and determined that breastfeeding is not the best choice for your family, there are healthful alter-natives, though you are not necessarily going to find them on the grocery store shelves. That being said, some formulas available in-store and online are going to be more healthful than others. You can find organic formulas that contain beneficial ingredients such as DHA and leave out the nasty stuff like corn syrup. Before deciding on any of these options, discuss the risks and benefits with your baby's pediatrician.

- **Homemade formula:** This method can be time intensive, but you can make it in larger batches and freeze it to save time. Sally Fallon, author of *Nourishing Traditions* and *The Nourishing Traditions Book of Baby &*

Child Care, has recipes in her books and online for dairy formula using cow or goat's milk and nondairy formula using beef or chicken broth and liver. These formulas are made with high-quality ingredients with a better nutritional profile than most commercial formulas.

- **Milk sharing:** There are organizations that help mothers obtain breast milk by connecting them with moms who have extra milk to donate, with no cost to either party (except possibly a fee to register with the organization). There are more milk-sharing programs popping up all the time, but MilkShare (*http://milkshare.birthingforlife.com*) and Human Milk 4 Human Babies (*www.hm4hb.net*) are two of the larger programs.
- **Milk banks:** These are similar to milk sharing, but milk donated to milk banks is pasteurized and tested for safety in a central location before being distributed to local milk banks. Under most circumstances, you have to pay out of pocket for this milk, but you may be able to receive at least partial reimbursement from your insurance company. To find a milk bank in your area, visit the Human Milk Banking Association of North America (*www.hmbana.org*).
- **Store-bought/Online:** When choosing a store-bought or online baby formula, be sure to carefully review the ingredient label. There are many options out there, with varying nutrient sources, but the best options will contain organic and natural ingredients. There are also allergy-friendly varieties if your baby has a dairy allergy.

The American Academy of Pediatrics (AAP) recommends exclusive breastfeeding for the first six months, with continued breastfeeding, along with solid foods, until at least your baby's first birthday. Any amount of breast milk you can give your baby is going to pass along health benefits. Even if you choose to breastfeed for only the first few days of your baby's life, or to give your baby a small amount of breast milk each day and supplement with other feeding methods, each and every drop will boost your child's growth and development.

Postpartum Recovery

Ever heard someone say that giving birth is more difficult than running a marathon? Most women who have been through labor and delivery will probably tell you that this is true, and that after accomplishing such an amazing physical, mental, and emotional feat, your body and mind will need time to bounce back. After giving birth, your baby becomes the center of your universe, but you can't forget to nurture yourself during this time, too. Your body is going through some pretty intense changes, and you need to take time to care for yourself with rest and a healthy diet to fully recover.

Postpartum Body Changes

Immediately after giving birth, you'll lose around ten pounds (sometimes less, sometimes more) because you are no longer carrying a baby or the placenta, and you'll lose some blood and amniotic fluid. Your body will probably be sore and tired all over from the stress and hard work of labor. Over the next few days and weeks, you will experience vaginal bleeding and discharge (called *lochia*) and menstrual-type cramps as your uterus shrinks to its pre-pregnancy size. If you had a vaginal birth, you'll probably have some pain and swelling. Unfortunately, if you suffered from constipation, hemorrhoids, and fatigue during pregnancy, they won't magically disappear overnight, and you may still experience some symptoms. Urinary incontinence is common, too, due to weakened pelvic floor muscles. Relaxin is still present in your body and your other hormones are shifting as well. Estrogen begins to drop while prolactin increases, and this can bring on mood swings, called the "baby blues," and contribute to temporary hair loss, breakouts, and excessive sweating.

A Healthy Lifestyle Is the Key to Recovery

With all of these changes, it will take time for your body to return to normal (or your new "normal"), but there are things you can do to encourage healing and boost your energy. On top of the fact that you just accomplished an astounding physical feat, sleep is hard to come by, so it's normal to feel tired and fatigued when caring for a newborn. Adding in small snacks between meals can keep energy levels on an even keel and ensure that you get the extra calories you need if you are breastfeeding. Foods high in potassium, such as bananas, dark leafy greens, fish, and avocados, can fight exhaustion by giving you an energy boost. The fiber in fruits and vegetables can alleviate constipation, and the complex carbohydrates keep your energy levels up, too, because they take a while to digest. Incorporating a mix of seafood, poultry, and red meat can guarantee that you get enough protein and iron to speed your recovery. Protein is super-important to aid in the rebuilding and repair of your body's tissues and to support your immune system, while iron-rich foods can help prevent anemia from loss of blood during and after childbirth. And keep guzzling down that water, too. Dehydration only exacerbates feelings of fatigue, and adequate water intake helps your body to distribute and use all those nutrients you are taking in.

ESSENTIAL

After a vaginal delivery, you can use witch hazel pads (available at most drug stores) to ease pain and promote healing. *Midwifery Today* suggests soaking a cloth in cold water, wringing it out, soaking it in witch hazel, and applying it to your perineum. You can also fill a spritz or peri bottle with a mixture of water and witch hazel.

There are practical measures you can take to help your body heal as well. While you are resting or sleeping, your body is working hard to repair itself. It can be hard to maximize rest time and sleep, but you can do a few things to make the transition easier for you and your baby:

- **Sleep when the baby sleeps:** Most mothers will tell you that they received this same advice and didn't follow it, but wish they had. You probably won't be able to sleep every time your baby is sleeping, but try to sneak in a nap here and there or let someone else watch over the baby while you snooze. If you prefer, you can bring your baby into bed with you to nurse. Even if you aren't asleep, you'll get to lie down and rest while your baby eats. Be sure to take the proper precautions for sleep-sharing just in case you do happen to fall asleep while your baby is in bed with you.
- **Take it easy:** If you've had a vaginal birth, most practitioners will give you the green light on physical activity and sexual intercourse after a six-week recovery period. Until then, short walks and light activity around the house should be okay. You may need more time, so it is crucial that you pay attention to your body and look for warning signs that you've jumped back in too quickly. If your bleeding increases or you pass any

clots or develop a fever, or if you experience persistent headaches, vomiting, or extreme fatigue, or if your pain and cramping don't seem to improve, contact your health care provider immediately.

- **Do Kegels:** You do need to limit physical activity until you get the go-ahead from your health care provider, but you should be able to start doing your Kegels right away. These exercises can help with urinary incontinence and speed the return of your pelvic floor muscles to their pre-pregnancy state.

- **Wear comfortable clothing:** You probably won't be wearing your pre-pregnancy clothes home from the hospital, but even if you can, you'll most likely be more comfortable in workout wear or pajamas than in your skinny jeans. Wear what feels comfortable for you. Especially if you are nursing, you'll want to wear special nursing tops or shirts that offer easy access for breastfeeding.

- **Take a shower:** Sometimes all you need is a five-minute shower to feel like a new woman! Steal a few minutes for yourself and take a rejuvenating bath or shower. A warm bath can be especially soothing if you experienced any tears during delivery or if you have hemorrhoids.

- **Go for a walk:** Most practitioners will give you the "thumbs up" to go for short daily walks just a few days after giving birth. Even a walk around the block will get you some fresh air and allow you to soak up some much-needed vitamin D. Bring your baby along in a stroller or baby carrier, or, if you need a breather, take a quiet walk on your own.

- **Let the house get a little messy:** There is a difference between messy and dirty. Let the mail stack up (but don't forget to pay your bills), forget about that pile of laundry that needs folding, and don't worry about the mess of toys on the living room floor. They will still be there after you've had that nap or a healthy snack.

- **Let family and friends help:** For many women, it is hard to ask for help, and it is easy to brush people off when they offer. Anyone who has been through what you've been through and offers to help *genuinely* wants to help, so let her. It can be something as simple as loading the dishwasher or picking up a few necessities from the grocery store on her way over. Let your friends bring you a nice hot meal and let your mom hold the baby so you can take that shower. Maybe you'll even have time to brush your teeth!

- **Keep often-used items nearby:** Remember that nursing caddy? Even if you aren't nursing, you will find it useful to keep a basket of regularly needed items nearby, such as your water bottle, phone charger, and lip balm. If you have stairs, you can even set up an area for diaper changes on each floor to limit going back and forth all day. A portable bassinet allows baby to sleep wherever you happen to be.

Recovery after a Cesarean

Your body needs extra special care after a cesarean delivery (C-section). A C-section is major abdominal surgery, so you may need pain relief medication and you'll probably have a longer hospital stay than someone who had a vaginal birth. You might feel sleepy and nauseated while you recover from anesthesia and surgery, and you'll need to care for your incision. You will still have lochia and cramping for a few weeks, but it may not be as heavy. On top of the healing methods you've already read, there are other considerations you need to make regarding your recovery.

QUESTION

What is a postpartum doula?
Most people think of a doula as someone who assists with labor and delivery, but there are postpartum doulas as well. A postpartum doula, as the name suggests, can help you out after the baby is born. She can care for you in a number of ways that will relieve a bit of postpartum stress and help you ease into motherhood, including running errands, offering breastfeeding tips, cooking meals, and feeding the baby.

- **Breastfeeding after a C-section:** If you choose to breastfeed, most facilities will allow you to nurse right after surgery. A nurse or lactation consultant can help you position the baby comfortably so that you don't irritate your incision.
- **Extra recovery time:** After a C-section, you need to give yourself extra time to recover. Not only are you recovering from abdominal surgery, you are also dealing with the demanding schedule of caring for a newborn. Once you return home, let someone bring the baby to you to nurse

(or let a friend or family member handle late-night bottle feedings) so you can rest as much as possible. A comfy pillow can support your achy back and, when you hold it against your stomach, soften the pain of coughing or sneezing. You will most likely be advised not to drive or do any heavy lifting for a few weeks following your surgery. Rest and relax as much as possible and take a few shortcuts in the kitchen, such as having freezer meals prepared before you give birth and making large meals in the slow cooker with lots of leftovers (e.g., Kitchen Sink Soup in Chapter 18 and Easy Peasy Beef Roast in Chapter 9). Even if you think you feel fine, follow your care provider's instructions regarding rest and physical activity. Expect a wait of between six and twelve weeks before you can resume exercise and sexual intercourse.

- **Incision care:** Your incision will take time to heal and your care provider will give you instructions on how to care for it properly. Avoid movements that can aggravate the incision, such as reaching overhead, lifting heavy items, and excessively bending or stretching. A Paleo diet can help with the healing process. Animal sources of protein support the repair and regeneration of cells after surgery, and the vitamins and fiber in fruits and vegetables are beneficial as well. Call your care provider immediately if you think your incision may be infected. Common signs of infection include a fever and warmth, redness, swelling, and/or oozing at the incision site.
- **Limited activity:** Even sitting up and walking will probably be uncomfortable for a while after your C-section, and it can take up to twelve weeks before you can resume your normal exercise routine. Even when resting, you can perform Kegels and gentle stretching exercises to tighten up your pelvic floor muscles and boost circulation. Before you leave the hospital, your practitioner will advise you to walk around to encourage blood flow and keep your digestive system moving, which will alleviate any gas and bloating. Continue with short daily walks after you return home to regain strength and stamina.

Postpartum Fitness

If you were an avid exerciser before and during pregnancy, you'll probably be itching to lace up your running shoes, but you need to make sure your body is ready and fully recovered before you begin an exercise routine. Your health care provider will give you the final word at your checkup, usually about six weeks postpartum, and you should then be free to jump back into your old routine or start a brand new one. Your practitioner will let you know of any restrictions you should be aware of. Once you do get your provider's consent, you'll want to start slow and ease back into your workout regimen. Even if you've been walking and doing your pelvic floor exercises daily, after a six-week (or longer) hiatus from strenuous physical activity, you may lose some level of fitness. So go easy on yourself if you can't lift the same amount of weight or find yourself huffing and puffing at the end of your spin class. It's more important that you take your time getting back into exercise to avoid injuries that may put you on the sidelines even longer.

ESSENTIAL

Many women experience aches and pains due to weakened core and lower back muscles after pregnancy. Throw that in with carrying around a baby all day and you might feel pretty uncomfortable by the end of the day. Yoga can gently stretch your body, while Pilates and other core and lower back–strengthening exercises can ease soreness and regain power.

You will still need water before, during, and after exercise to keep from getting dehydrated, and a meal or small snack about an hour before working out. If your workout will be longer than an hour, throw in an easy-to-digest snack, such as a small piece of fruit, around the sixty-minute mark. Don't forget your post-workout recovery meal (refer to Chapter 5) to get your muscles on the fast track to recovery. Remember, if you are breastfeeding, you should already be taking in extra calories. When working out, you need to make sure you are eating enough to support your milk supply.

There are warning signs that you should look out for when you begin exercising again. If you feel faint or dizzy, have an increase in vaginal bleeding, or experience pain or cramping, stop exercising immediately. If your condition doesn't improve, call your health care provider or emergency services.

The big question you are probably asking yourself is how to find the time to exercise. It might seem as if your world has been turned upside down and you can't find a minute for yourself, but there are ways to incorporate fitness into your daily routine. Many gyms offer childcare as part of your membership or for a small additional fee. You can also sneak in an early morning or late evening workout when the baby is sleeping, or when you have a friend or family member who can take over for a bit. No extra hands to hold your bundle of joy while you exercise? Bring baby along with you! If you are a runner, check with your pediatrician to find out when you can safely run with your baby in a running stroller (you'll want to make sure that your baby has good head and neck control first). Most cities have walking groups, yoga studios, and fitness classes available where you can work out with your baby and meet other moms. There are also exercise videos specifically designed for moms and babies. Your baby just became the cutest dumbbell in history!

QUESTION

Is it safe to lose weight while breastfeeding?
When it comes to postpartum weight loss while breastfeeding, slow and steady wins the race. If you cut too many calories or work out too intensely, your milk supply can suffer. By sticking to a Paleo diet of whole foods and exercising regularly, you'll lose weight gradually without hurting your supply.

Realities of Postpartum Depression and Anxiety

Strong emotions are totally normal after having a baby. You can be crying tears of joy one minute and shedding tears of sadness over the loss of your old life the next. Most women even experience a period of mild depression, the baby blues, that can last anywhere from a couple of days to a couple of weeks. There are various reasons you may feel a little down and out after giving birth—exhaustion, lack of sleep, changing hormone levels, a disappointing birth experience, and anxiety over properly caring for your baby, just to name a few. The baby blues do not require treatment and will go away on their own once you begin to adjust to motherhood.

Symptoms of Postpartum Depression

Sometimes the baby blues don't resolve on their own, signaling a more serious problem such as postpartum depression or postpartum anxiety. While they do share some similarities and it is possible to suffer from both, postpartum depression and postpartum anxiety are two separate conditions. Symptoms of postpartum depression include the following:

- Feelings of extreme sadness or anger
- Loss of interest in your favorite activities or spending time with loved ones
- Changes in appetite
- Trouble sleeping when your baby sleeps
- Lack of energy
- Difficulty concentrating or making decisions
- Feelings of low self-esteem
- Suicidal thoughts
- Feeling disconnected from your baby
- Having thoughts about hurting your baby
- Feeling guilty about not being able to properly care for your baby

Source: The Centers for Disease Control: Depression Among Women of Reproductive Age

ALERT

Postpartum psychosis is a rare but serious condition that requires urgent medical treatment. Symptoms include delusions, hallucinations, inability to sleep, rapid mood swings, difficulty communicating, hyperactivity, and attempting to hurt yourself or your baby. Seek immediate medical attention if you think you may be suffering from postpartum psychosis. It is possible for any woman to develop postpartum psychosis, but you are at greater risk if you have a severe mental illness such as schizophrenia or bipolar disorder, or have a family history of either of these conditions.

Symptoms of postpartum anxiety include the following:

- Constantly worrying or anxious about your baby's health
- Feelings of intense worry or panic (panic attacks)
- Physical symptoms such as shortness of breath, chest pain, dizziness, and hot flashes

While the exact causes are not known, postpartum depression and anxiety, which affect about 10–18 percent of new mothers, are often attributed to hormonal, environmental, and physiological factors, as well as genetic predisposition. If you suffered from depression or anxiety before or during pregnancy, you may be at a greater risk. It is critical that you see your health care provider if you are experiencing any of the symptoms listed here.

Treatment for Postpartum Depression

Postpartum depression can be treated with counseling and/or medication. Your health care provider can refer you to a specialist who will find the right treatment for you. There are things you can do to cope and care for yourself, as well, to help prevent and treat postpartum depression and anxiety:

- **Supportive foods:** While diet alone cannot treat depression, it can help to prevent and alleviate symptoms. An overall diet rich in vitamins, minerals, and antioxidants has a protective effect on the body and reduces free radical damage, the process by which certain molecules in the body damage the DNA of other cells and interfere with normal function, which can lead to disease. Protein, carbohydrates, and healthy fats support the growth and repair of tissues and keep your body running at top potential. On top of that, many recent studies have proven a link between certain nutrient deficiencies and an increased risk for depression. A 2005 study published in *Biological Psychology* showed that deficiencies of omega-3 fatty acids, folate, vitamin B_{12}, iron, zinc, and selenium are more common among women who develop postpartum depression than those who do not. This could be due in part to nutrient reserves being depleted during pregnancy and lactation—all the more reason to consume a high-quality, nutrient-dense diet before, during, and after pregnancy.

- **Exercise:** There are a number of ways that regular exercise can help to prevent and treat depression. Fresh air, sunshine (and the vitamin D that comes along with it), and quality time on a walk with friends can definitely make you feel better and give you an energy boost when you are feeling down, but it is actually scientifically proven that exercise is an effective way to treat depression. First of all, the endorphins released during exercise can amp up your mood and lessen pain. Studies also show a connection between moderate physical activity (even as little as 20–30 minutes per day) and a decreased risk of developing depression throughout life.

- **Support system:** Having a strong support system in place can be beneficial on many fronts. Having loved ones to care for your baby, help with household chores, and confide in can alleviate some of the stress of being a new mom. There are also support groups available, both local and online, for mothers who suffer from postpartum depression. Visit Postpartum Support International (*www.postpartum.net*) for resources in your area.

- **Self-care:** It's essential that you continue to care for yourself and meet even your most basic needs, like showering, painting your nails, or throwing on an outfit you feel great in. Doing something small that is just for you can really help to lift your spirits.

- **Rest and relaxation:** Even if you can't sleep, take a break from the day and relax. Read a book or lie down when your baby is sleeping. Don't feel bad if things around the house are left undone. Focus on yourself and your baby and the rest will fall into place.

ALERT

Although some drugs are contraindicated for breastfeeding, there are certain drugs that treat depression and are considered safe for breastfeeding. The dangers of leaving depression untreated are greater than the small amount of medication that you may pass to the baby through your breast milk. Speak with your practitioner about which antidepressant medications are recommended for breastfeeding women.

Adjusting to Your New Reality

No matter how much you prepare, adjusting to life with a newborn can really throw you for a loop. You are now a mother with a tiny person to care for, but that isn't all you are. You are still the same strong, beautiful woman you were before giving birth, and it is possible to integrate who you were with who you are now and who you want to become. Your body might not look exactly the same, and some of your priorities may change, but you will find time for the things you've always loved and will probably even make some new friends along the way while you learn to maneuver your new life as "Mommy."

Shifting Priorities

When you bring home your baby, you bring home a whole new set of priorities along with him. Keeping your family (yourself included) healthy and happy is probably at the top of your list and that may mean shifting your expectations in other areas.

For example:

- Try not to worry about the little things and lighten your load when you can. Accept a friend or family member's offer to come by to help you clean the house . . . or just forget about vacuuming until next week.
- If someone wants to come by, ask her to check in with you before she heads over in case you are having a rough day and would rather nap than entertain visitors.
- Order in a healthy Paleo meal from a local restaurant if you don't have the time or energy to cook a meal.
- Most of all, go with the flow. Even if you have a plan for the day, your baby may have a different one, so you need to be ready to throw your plan out the window and roll with the punches.

It Takes a Village

You've probably heard it said that it takes a village to raise a child. We may not live in small, close-knit communities anymore, but that doesn't mean you can't form your own village. Lean on family and friends for emotional support, childcare, and help with daily activities. Join a new moms' support group to meet other women who are experiencing the same things that you are. You can share all the joyous "firsts" of being a new mom, and you can also find comfort in knowing that you aren't alone in your frustration and uncertainty about motherhood.

ESSENTIAL

Most communities have groups for new moms that give babies a chance to socialize (depending on their ages) and moms a chance to laugh, cry, and commiserate with other new moms. You may make new lifelong friends and find a few new playmates for your little one. Many groups even have speakers come in to cover various topics, such as baby sign language, introducing solid foods, and baby yoga. Check with your local baby stores, practitioner, hospital, or birthing center for groups in your area.

Making Time for a Healthy Lifestyle

Parenthood can seem overwhelming at first, but as you fall into your new routine, you will find ways to make it work for you, all while integrating your healthy Paleo lifestyle. Sleep and free time may be hard to come by, but there are ways to best use the time you do have to maximize nutrition, exercise, and rest.

- Make a large salad on Sunday that you can eat for lunch over the next few days, instead of urgently trying to make a meal when your baby is hungry and crying. Better yet, slip your baby into a baby carrier and cuddle with her while you prepare your meal (being careful not to get too close to the stove or oven).
- Always make enough for leftovers and refrigerate or freeze them for later use. The Mini Denver Omelets (see Chapter 7) freeze perfectly! Make a double batch and save the extras for a busy morning.
- Make a super-simple breakfast of berries and a couple of hard-boiled eggs.

- Sleep when your baby is sleeping. Your sleep may be broken up into short spurts throughout the day, but try to get in some shuteye whenever you can.
- Spread exercise out over the course of the day. If you can only manage ten minutes here and there, do what you can and watch it add up throughout the day!
- Exercise with your baby in the stroller. Try walking lunges while pushing the stroller or let baby face you and watch you while you do pushups, squats, or sit-ups.

Your Amazing New Body

You might be zipping up your pre-pregnancy jeans just a few weeks after giving birth, or you might still feel more comfortable in your maternity jeans. The good news is . . . it doesn't matter one bit. Your body has just done something amazing, some might even say miraculous. Over the past nine months, your body has created and nurtured a human life, and now you are working even harder to care for that little baby here in the real world. That is something to be proud of, no matter your size or the pregnancy battle wounds (i.e., stretch marks, sagging breasts, and a little extra belly) you earned along the way.

We are all different and so are our bodies. Slow and steady weight loss is the way to go post-baby to minimize emotional and physical stress. If you have certain weight-loss or strength objectives that you want to achieve, set realistic goals and give yourself a reasonable timeline to meet those goals. The truth is, your body may never look quite the same, and that is okay. The important thing is that you take care of yourself and your family, and you are well on your way to doing that by following a nutrient-dense, whole-foods, Paleo way of living.

CHAPTER 7

Hearty Breakfasts and Brunches

Banana Pancakes

Giving up grains doesn't mean giving up pancakes. These pancakes are naturally sweetened with bananas. Perfect for Sunday morning brunch!

INGREDIENTS | SERVES 2

2 ripe medium bananas, mashed

3 large eggs

½ teaspoon vanilla extract

2 tablespoons coconut flour

½ teaspoon cinnamon

¼ teaspoon nutmeg

⅛ teaspoon sea salt

½ teaspoon baking powder

1 tablespoon coconut oil

Toppings Galore!

When it comes to pancake toppings, there are endless options. Try fresh or sautéed berries, pure maple syrup, raisins, sliced bananas, a dash of cinnamon, or even a dollop of almond butter.

1. Heat a large skillet or griddle pan over medium heat.

2. Add bananas, eggs, and vanilla to a high-powered blender. Blend until well combined. Add coconut flour, cinnamon, nutmeg, salt, and baking powder to blender. Blend until smooth.

3. Evenly grease skillet or griddle pan with coconut oil. Pour batter onto pan, making silver dollar–sized pancakes.

4. Cook for 2–3 minutes until pancakes start to bubble and the edges turn a golden brown. Flip and cook for an additional 2–3 minutes. Repeat with remaining batter.

PER SERVING Calories: 346 | Fat: 22g | Protein: 12g | Sodium: 375mg | Fiber: 8g | Carbohydrates: 33g | Sugar: 15g

Garden Veggie Omelet

This protein-packed dish wraps up fresh vegetables with light, fluffy eggs and is the perfect breakfast boost for when you're feeling tired or low on energy.

INGREDIENTS | SERVES 2

1 teaspoon ghee or coconut oil
4 large eggs
1 tablespoon water
⅛ teaspoon sea salt
⅛ teaspoon pepper
1 cup chopped spinach
6 cherry tomatoes, halved
1 green onion, diced

1. Heat a medium nonstick skillet over medium heat. Once hot, add ghee or coconut oil to pan.

2. Crack eggs into a medium bowl. Add water, salt, and pepper. Whisk well.

3. Pour eggs into pan. When eggs begin to set around the edges, use a spatula to push cooked eggs toward the center of the pan, and tilt skillet so the uncooked eggs can spread to the bottom of the skillet.

4. When eggs are almost set, sprinkle spinach, cherry tomatoes, and green onion evenly over half of the omelet.

5. Use a spatula to fold the omelet in half. Cook for 2 minutes, until eggs are fully cooked.

PER SERVING Calories: 177 | Fat: 12g | Protein: 14g | Sodium: 300mg | Fiber: 1g | Carbohydrates: 4g | Sugar: 2g

Sweet Potato and Bacon Hash

This is a sweet and savory veggie-filled breakfast hash that will get you going and keep you satisfied all morning long! Add a side of scrambled eggs for even more staying power.

INGREDIENTS | SERVES 2

2 slices bacon
½ medium yellow onion, diced
1 medium sweet potato, grated
½ teaspoon paprika
½ teaspoon cinnamon
⅛ teaspoon sea salt
⅛ teaspoon pepper

Feed the Whole Family

This recipe makes two servings, but it can be easily doubled or even tripled to feed a large group. If you want to experiment with different flavors, try swapping in cumin and chili powder for the paprika and cinnamon and adding ½ cup of diced bell pepper for a taste of the Southwest. You can also add a grated zucchini and spice with rosemary and thyme for a garden herb flavor.

1. Add bacon to a large cold skillet and heat over medium heat. Cook until evenly browned and just beginning to crisp, flipping often, 7–10 minutes. Remove to a paper towel–lined plate and set aside.

2. Add onion to the same pan and cook until translucent, stirring often, 3–5 minutes.

3. Add grated sweet potato and spices to the pan and stir well to combine. Cook until softened, 8–10 minutes.

4. Once bacon has cooled, roughly chop and return to pan with onion and sweet potato. Stir well to combine before serving.

PER SERVING Calories: 170 | Fat: 10g | Protein: 4g | Sodium: 370mg | Fiber: 2g | Carbohydrates: 16g | Sugar: 4g

Mini Denver Omelets

These bite-sized omelets are perfect when you are on the go. Grab a couple for breakfast or a snack, and you are out the door with your new baby in tow!

INGREDIENTS | SERVES 4

1½ tablespoons ghee

2 medium green bell peppers, seeded and diced

½ medium yellow onion, diced

8 large eggs

⅛ teaspoon sea salt

⅛ teaspoon pepper

4 slices organic deli ham, diced

Make-Ahead for Postpartum Breakfasts

These mini omelets are a great make-ahead breakfast option when you are short on time. They will keep for 5 days in the refrigerator or 2 to 3 months in the freezer in an airtight container. When you are ready to eat, place the mini omelets directly in the microwave to reheat until warmed, about 1½ minutes.

1. Preheat oven to 350°F. Grease a 12-muffin tin with ½ tablespoon ghee or use a silicon muffin pan.

2. Heat remaining ghee in a large skillet over medium heat. Add the bell pepper and onion and sauté until softened, stirring often, 5–7 minutes. Remove from heat.

3. In a large bowl, beat eggs with salt and pepper. Stir in diced ham, and cooked onion and bell pepper.

4. Use a small measuring cup to spoon mixture evenly into the muffin cups. Bake for 20–25 minutes, until eggs are set and just beginning to brown on top.

PER SERVING Calories: 248 | Fat: 17g | Protein: 18g | Sodium: 580mg | Fiber: 2g | Carbohydrates: 6g | Sugar: 3g

Ginger Carrot Breakfast Casserole

Paleo breakfasts are often savory dishes, but the apples and spices lend a subtle sweetness to this hearty breakfast casserole. This dish also freezes well for easy reheating on busy mornings.

INGREDIENTS | SERVES 6

2 tablespoons coconut oil
½ large white onion, diced
4 large carrots, peeled and grated
1 medium apple, peeled and grated
1 teaspoon cinnamon
½ teaspoon nutmeg
½ teaspoon ginger
¼ teaspoon allspice
¼ teaspoon sea salt, divided
¼ teaspoon pepper, divided
½ pound ground pork
8 large eggs

1. Preheat oven to 425°F.

2. Heat coconut oil in a large skillet over medium heat. Add onion and cook until translucent, stirring frequently, about 3 minutes.

3. Add carrots and apple to skillet. Cook for an additional 5 minutes, stirring occasionally. Stir in cinnamon, nutmeg, ginger, allspice, ⅛ teaspoon salt, and ⅛ teaspoon pepper.

4. Add ground pork and cook until browned, using a spatula to break it up and incorporate it as it cooks.

5. Meanwhile, in a large bowl, beat the eggs with remaining salt and pepper.

6. Transfer pork mixture from the skillet to a 9" × 13" glass baking dish and pour eggs evenly over the top. Use a fork to incorporate eggs with carrot mixture. Bake for 25–30 minutes, until eggs are cooked through.

PER SERVING Calories: 270 | Fat: 19g | Protein: 15g | Sodium: 245mg | Fiber: 2g | Carbohydrates: 9g | Sugar: 6g

Zesty Italian Brunch Bake

The roasted red peppers and spices in this vegetable-packed dish provide its signature "zest" without making it too spicy.

INGREDIENTS | SERVES 4

3 large jarred roasted red peppers, sliced in half lengthwise

½ large yellow onion, thinly sliced

1 medium zucchini, thinly sliced

6 button mushrooms, sliced

½ pound ground beef

6 large eggs

1 teaspoon oregano

1 teaspoon parsley

1 teaspoon garlic powder

⅛ teaspoon sea salt

⅛ teaspoon pepper

1. Preheat oven to 350°F.

2. If peppers are stored in oil, rinse and pat dry with a paper towel to soak up any excess moisture. Line the bottom of an 8" × 8" glass baking dish with sliced peppers.

3. Sprinkle onions on top of peppers. Layer zucchini slices over onions. Place mushroom slices over zucchini.

4. Heat a large skillet over medium heat. Add ground beef and cook until browned, 7–10 minutes. Drain fat from beef, and pour beef into the baking dish, evenly covering mushrooms.

5. In a large bowl, beat eggs with oregano, parsley, garlic powder, salt, and pepper. Pour evenly into the baking dish and shake it around a bit to make sure everything is evenly covered.

6. Bake for 45–50 minutes, until eggs are cooked through.

PER SERVING Calories: 238 | Fat: 13g | Protein: 23g | Sodium: 224mg | Fiber: 1g | Carbohydrates: 7g | Sugar: 5g

Scrambled Eggs and Chicken Sausage

This is a great simple breakfast for those mornings when you haven't had a lot of sleep!
Add a side of fresh berries or sliced banana for a quick and easy breakfast.

INGREDIENTS | SERVES 2

1 tablespoon coconut oil

2 chicken sausage links, sliced

4 large eggs

⅛ teaspoon sea salt

⅛ teaspoon pepper

Check the Label

When shopping for Paleo chicken sausage, be sure to read the label. Look for nitrate-free chicken sausage without any sugar or artificial additives and preservatives.

1. Heat coconut oil in a large skillet over medium heat. Add sliced chicken sausage and cook undisturbed for 3–4 minutes, until browned on one side.

2. While sausage is cooking, beat the eggs in a medium bowl with salt and pepper. Flip chicken sausage to brown other side. After 1 minute, pour the eggs into the pan with the chicken sausage and stir until eggs are fully cooked, about 5 minutes.

PER SERVING Calories: 368 | Fat: 26g | Protein: 33g | Sodium: 846mg | Fiber: 0g | Carbohydrates: 1g | Sugar: 1g

Fried Apple and Eggs

Fruit and scrambled eggs may seem like an unlikely combination, but this sweet and creamy egg scramble will surprise you!

INGREDIENTS | SERVES 2

1 tablespoon coconut oil

1 medium MacIntosh apple, thinly sliced and peeled (if you prefer)

½ teaspoon cinnamon

¼ teaspoon nutmeg

4 large eggs

¼ cup coconut milk

¼ teaspoon vanilla

⅛ teaspoon sea salt

⅛ teaspoon pepper

1. Heat coconut oil in a large skillet over medium heat. Add apple slices, cinnamon, and nutmeg and cook for about 5 minutes, stirring often, until softened.

2. While apples are cooking, beat eggs in a medium bowl with coconut milk, vanilla, salt, and pepper.

3. Evenly pour the eggs into the pan with the apple slices and stir until eggs are fully cooked, about 5 minutes.

PER SERVING Calories: 297 | Fat: 23g | Protein: 13g | Sodium: 290mg | Fiber: 1g | Carbohydrates: 12g | Sugar: 9g

Roasted Brussels Sprouts and Butternut Squash

This warming breakfast is perfect for a cool, fall morning. It's also great as a side dish to roasted pork or a whole roasted chicken.

INGREDIENTS | SERVES 4

1 pound Brussels sprouts, trimmed and halved

1 small butternut squash, peeled, seeded, and cut into ½" cubes

1 medium yellow onion, diced

2 tablespoons coconut oil

⅛ teaspoon sea salt

⅛ teaspoon pepper

2 tablespoons dried cranberries (no sugar or oil added)

1. Preheat oven to 425°F.

2. In a large bowl, toss Brussels sprouts, butternut squash, and onion with coconut oil, salt, and pepper until everything is evenly coated.

3. Spread vegetables onto a large rimmed baking sheet. Roast for 40–45 minutes, stirring after 20 minutes. Remove from oven when vegetables are tender and beginning to brown. Stir in dried cranberries and serve warm.

PER SERVING Calories: 178 | Fat: 7g | Protein: 5g | Sodium: 107mg | Fiber: 7g | Carbohydrates: 28g | Sugar: 8g

Zucchini and Spinach Breakfast

This breakfast is full of good-for-you greens with a punch of flavor thanks to the minced garlic.

INGREDIENTS | SERVES 4

2 slices bacon
1 medium yellow onion, diced
2 cloves garlic, minced
4 medium zucchini, grated
½ cup julienne cut sun-dried tomatoes
2 cups baby spinach, roughly chopped

Did You Know?

Spinach is a good source of folate, one of the most important nutrients you need during pregnancy. Folate is necessary for the proper development of the neural tube, and the spinach in this breakfast can help you meet your daily goal.

1. Add bacon to a large cold skillet and heat over medium heat. Cook until evenly browned and just beginning to crisp, flipping often, about 7–10 minutes. Remove to a paper towel–lined plate and set aside. Crumble bacon once cooled.

2. Add onion and garlic to skillet and cook, stirring often, until fragrant, about 3 minutes.

3. Add zucchini and sun-dried tomatoes to skillet and cook, stirring occasionally, until zucchini is tender, about 5 minutes. Stir in spinach and cook until wilted, about 1 minute.

4. Divide vegetables evenly between 4 plates and top each plate with crumbled bacon.

PER SERVING Calories: 119 | Fat: 6g | Protein: 5g | Sodium: 265mg | Fiber: 4g | Carbohydrates: 14g | Sugar: 9g

Cinnamon-Spiced Apple Butter

If you're using a less tart apple, add the honey ¼ cup at a time, until you reach desired sweetness. Serve over a Paleo muffin or breakfast casserole.

INGREDIENTS | YIELDS 6 (½ CUP) SERVINGS

8 large or 12 medium Granny Smith apples

½ cup apple juice (fresh or 100% juice, no sugar added)

¾ cup honey

2 teaspoons ground cinnamon

½ teaspoon allspice

½ teaspoon ground cloves

1. Wash, peel, core, and quarter the apples. Add to a 2-quart slow cooker along with the juice. Cover and cook on high for 4 hours.

2. Use an immersion blender to purée the apples. Stir in the honey, cinnamon, allspice, and cloves. Taste for seasoning and adjust if necessary.

3. Reduce the temperature of the slow cooker to low. Cook uncovered for 2 hours or until the apple butter is thick and dark. Store in the refrigerator for up to 2 weeks or freeze until needed.

PER SERVING Calories: 141 | Fat: 0g | Protein: 0g | Sodium: 3mg | Fiber: 1g | Carbohydrates: 38g | Sugar: 37g

Ginger Tea

Ginger has been used for many years in Chinese medicine. It helps treat stomach pain, diarrhea, and morning sickness. You could also add honey or lemon juice to this tea for a delightful flavor.

INGREDIENTS | SERVES 4

2–3 pieces of gingerroot

4 cups cold water

1. Peel the ginger root and slice it into thin diagonal slices.

2. Boil water and add the ginger slices.

3. Simmer for 15 minutes, then strain the tea.

PER SERVING Calories: 30 | Fat: 0g | Protein: 0g | Sodium: 0mg | Carbohydrates: 8g | Sugar: 8g

CHAPTER 8

Appetizers, Dips, and Spreads

Classic Guacamole

The omega-3 fatty acids in avocado make this guacamole a pregnancy superfood. Serve over eggs, burgers, or salad, or enjoy it as a snack with veggie sticks or plantain chips.

INGREDIENTS | YIELDS 2 CUPS; SERVING SIZE: ½ CUP

2 medium avocados

2 tablespoons finely diced red onion

Juice of ½ medium lime

1 jalapeño, stem and seeds removed, finely diced

½ medium tomato, chopped

2 tablespoons roughly chopped fresh cilantro leaves

⅛ teaspoon sea salt

⅛ teaspoon pepper

1. Cut avocados in half and remove pits. Scoop avocado flesh into a large bowl and roughly mash with a fork.

2. Use fork to stir in remaining ingredients until well combined.

3. Serve immediately or press plastic wrap directly over the guacamole and store in an airtight container. Guacamole should last 1–2 days in the refrigerator.

PER SERVING Calories: 167 | Fat: 15g | Protein: 2g | Sodium: 83mg | Fiber: 7g | Carbohydrates: 10g | Sugar: 1.5g

A Taste of the Tropics

Transform this traditional guacamole into a tropical treat by adding diced mango. Mix up the guacamole per the instructions and stir in about ¼ cup of mango before serving.

Eggplant Dip (Baba Ghanoush)

Baba ghanoush is a traditional Middle Eastern eggplant spread. It is usually served with bread, but for Paleo folks it also makes a fantastic dip for veggie sticks.

INGREDIENTS | YIELDS 1½ CUPS; SERVING SIZE: ½ CUP

1 large eggplant
2½ tablespoons olive oil, divided
¼ teaspoon sea salt, divided
¼ teaspoon pepper, divided
1 clove garlic
2 tablespoons tahini (sesame seed paste)
Juice of ½ large lemon

1. Preheat oven to 450°F. Cut eggplant in half lengthwise and place cut side up on a large foil-lined baking dish. Prick the skin of each half a few times with a fork. Drizzle 1 tablespoon of olive oil over each half and sprinkle with ⅛ teaspoon each salt and pepper. Roast for 35–40 minutes, until tender. Remove from oven and allow to cool to room temperature.

2. Once cool, scoop the eggplant flesh into the bowl of a food processor. Add remaining salt and pepper, garlic, tahini, and lemon juice to food processor and process until smooth. Finish with a drizzle of the remaining ½ tablespoon of olive oil. Serve immediately or refrigerate in an airtight container for up to 1 week.

PER SERVING Calories: 165 | Fat: 12g | Protein: 4g | Sodium: 210mg | Fiber: 7g | Carbohydrates: 13g | Sugar: 4g

Tropical Fruit Salsa

A deliciously fruity summertime treat! Scoop it up with green apple slices or serve over fish or chicken.

**INGREDIENTS | YIELDS 2 CUPS;
SERVING SIZE: ½ CUP**

½ pineapple, cored and cut into large chunks

1 mango, peeled and cut into large chunks

½ medium red onion, roughly chopped

½ cup loosely packed fresh cilantro leaves

Juice of 1 medium lime

⅛ teaspoon sea salt

⅛ teaspoon pepper

Add all ingredients to food processor with the chopping blade attached. Pulse a few times until well combined and coarsely chopped. Serve immediately or store in an airtight container in the refrigerator for up to 5 days.

PER SERVING Calories: 97 | Fat: 0g | Protein: 1g | Sodium: 78mg | Fiber: 3g | Carbohydrates: 25g | Sugar: 19g

Spice It Up!
Kick the heat up a notch by adding smoky, sweet chipotle pepper to this salsa. Add 1 canned chipotle pepper in adobo sauce to food processor with other ingredients.

Stuffed Button Mushrooms

Perfect for a party appetizer or just as a fun snack, this delicious dish is sure to please all of your guests. Once you have the basic recipe down, you can switch it up by using different types of sausage and various herbs and spices.

INGREDIENTS | SERVES 8 AS AN APPETIZER

20 large button mushrooms

2 tablespoons olive oil

½ pound ground Italian sausage

½ medium white onion, finely diced

2 garlic cloves, minced

1 large egg, beaten

¼ cup almond meal

⅛ teaspoon sea salt

⅛ teaspoon pepper

1 teaspoon dried basil

1 teaspoon dried oregano

1. Preheat oven to 350°F. Remove stems from mushrooms; dice stems and set aside.

2. Place mushroom caps in a large bowl and toss with olive oil. Place mushroom caps in a large glass baking dish.

3. Heat a large skillet over medium heat. Once hot, add sausage and cook until it begins to brown, about 3–4 minutes. Stir with a spatula as it cooks to break up sausage.

4. Add onions, garlic, and diced mushroom stems to the pan. Cook, stirring occasionally, until vegetables are softened and sausage is fully cooked. Pour contents of pan into a large bowl. Stir in egg, almond meal, and spices.

5. Spoon a heaping tablespoon of the sausage mixture into each mushroom cap. Bake for 20–25 minutes. Turn heat up to broil and bake for an additional 3 minutes, until tops are brown and a nice crust forms. Remove from oven and let cool for 5 minutes before serving.

PER SERVING Calories: 155 | Fat: 13g | Protein: 7g | Sodium: 225mg | Fiber: 1g | Carbohydrates: 3g | Sugar: 1g

Fruit Kebabs

These rainbow-colored skewers are a fun and unique way to serve fruit.
It doesn't get much easier than this.

INGREDIENTS | SERVES 8

8 long wooden skewers

16 purple grapes

16 blueberries

16 green grapes

2 medium bananas, cut into 8 slices each

8 mandarin orange segments

16 raspberries

Thread fruit onto skewers in the order listed. Serve immediately or refrigerate, covered, for no longer than 2–3 hours.

PER SERVING Calories: 48 | Fat: 0g | Protein: 0g | Sodium: 1mg | Fiber: 1g | Carbohydrates: 12g | Sugar: 8g

Eat the Rainbow!

Various phytonutrients provide fruits (and vegetables) with their pigments. By eating a rainbow of brightly colored produce, you'll be consuming many different phytonutrients and soaking up the health benefits.

Paleo Mayonnaise

Most store-bought mayonnaise contains sugar, soybean oil, and chemical preservatives, while this homemade recipe contains only six healthy ingredients.

**INGREDIENTS | YIELDS 1½ CUPS;
SERVING SIZE:
2 TABLESPOONS**

2 large egg yolks, room temperature

2 teaspoons Dijon mustard (check the label for additives)

Juice of ½ large lemon

⅛ teaspoon sea salt

⅛ teaspoon pepper

1 cup olive oil

A Shortcut to Homemade Mayo

If you have an immersion blender, you can make this recipe even easier. Just add all ingredients except for the olive oil into the immersion blender cup. Pour olive oil on top. Insert immersion blender all the way to the bottom of the cup and turn it on, slowly tilting and lifting the head of the blender until all oil is emulsified.

1. Add egg yolks, mustard, lemon juice, salt, and pepper to a blender. Blend on low until well combined.

2. Very slowly add the olive oil while still blending on a low setting. Start adding the oil drop by drop. As the mixture emulsifies, you can gradually pour the oil in faster. Once all of the olive oil has been added, the mayonnaise should be a thick consistency. Store in the refrigerator in an airtight container for up to 2 weeks.

PER SERVING Calories: 169 | Fat: 19g | Protein: 1g | Sodium: 36mg | Fiber: 0g | Carbohydrates: 0g | Sugar: 0g

Spinach and Artichoke Dip

Most spinach and artichoke dips found in restaurants are not Paleo friendly because of the dairy and hydrogenated oils. You can whip this version up for a pre-dinner appetizer with vegetable sticks or spread it over fish or chicken before roasting.

INGREDIENTS | YIELDS 2 CUPS; SERVING SIZE: ½ CUP

6 ounces chopped frozen spinach, thawed and drained

14 ounces canned artichoke hearts, rinsed and drained

½ large avocado, peeled

1 garlic clove, minced

2 tablespoons chopped fresh basil

2 tablespoons lemon juice

1 teaspoon paprika

⅛ teaspoon sea salt

⅛ teaspoon pepper

1 medium roasted red pepper, diced

1. Place all ingredients except roasted red pepper into a food processor with the chopping blade attached. Pulse to combine until desired consistency is reached.

2. Stir in diced red pepper. Place in refrigerator to chill before serving. Store in an airtight container for up to 4 days in the refrigerator.

PER SERVING Calories: 103 | Fat: 4g | Protein: 5g | Sodium: 200mg | Fiber: 8g | Carbohydrates: 15g | Sugar: 2g

Bacon-Wrapped Dates

These salty-sweet goodies won't last long, and they will make your house smell amazing.

INGREDIENTS | SERVES 8 AS AN APPETIZER

1 teaspoon coconut oil

16 raw almonds

16 pitted Medjool dates

8 slices of bacon, cut in half width-wise

A Sweet Treat

Enjoy this sweet treat in moderation. Dates do have a high level of sweetness, but they also provide vitamins and minerals that you won't find in candy bars or baked goods.

1. Preheat oven to 400°F. Line a baking sheet with aluminum foil and place a wire cooling rack on top of the baking sheet. Brush or spray rack with coconut oil.

2. Stuff an almond inside of each date. Wrap each date with a half-slice of bacon. Place dates seam side down on the wire rack. Bake for 20–25 minutes until bacon is crispy.

PER SERVING Calories: 169 | Fat: 12g | Protein: 4g | Sodium: 189mg | Fiber: 1.5g | Carbohydrates: 13g | Sugar: 11g

Paleo Pesto

This delicious pesto recipe utilizes fresh ingredients for fabulous flavor and maximum health benefits. You can keep it in the refrigerator for 2–3 days, and in the freezer for up to 1 month.

INGREDIENTS | YIELDS 3 CUPS; SERVING SIZE: ¼ CUP

2 cups baby spinach leaves, washed and dried

1 cup fresh basil leaves, washed and dried

½ cup toasted unsalted pine nuts

6 garlic cloves, peeled

2 tablespoons lemon juice

1 cup extra-virgin olive oil, divided

1 teaspoon sea salt

1 teaspoon freshly ground black pepper

1. In a food processor, combine the spinach, basil, pine nuts, garlic cloves, lemon juice, and ¼ cup of the olive oil. Process until well blended.

2. Continue blending while drizzling in remaining olive oil until desired consistency is achieved.

3. Add sea salt and pepper and pulse to combine.

PER SERVING Calories: 223 | Fat: 24g | Protein: 2g | Sodium: 209mg | Fiber: 1g | Carbohydrates: 3g | Sugar: 0.1g

CHAPTER 9

Beef, Lamb, and Pork

Lettuce-Wrapped Bison Burgers

Without the bun, hamburgers make for a totally customizable Paleo meal that can be eaten for breakfast, lunch, or dinner.

INGREDIENTS | SERVES 4

1 pound ground bison
¼ teaspoon sea salt
½ teaspoon black pepper
¼ teaspoon garlic powder
1 tablespoon ghee
4 large leaves of iceberg lettuce
1 medium tomato, sliced
½ small red onion, thinly sliced
Optional toppings: bacon, pickles, Classic Guacamole (see recipe in Chapter 8), mustard, Paleo Mayonnaise (see recipe in Chapter 8), salsa, etc.

1. In a large bowl, combine ground bison, salt, pepper, and garlic powder. Form 4 patties and lay flat on a plate.

2. Heat ghee in a large skillet or grill pan over medium-high heat. Place burgers in skillet and cook, undisturbed, for 5 minutes. Flip burgers and cook for an additional 5 minutes, or to your desired level of doneness.

3. Place each burger on a lettuce leaf. Top with sliced tomato, red onion, and any additional toppings before you finish wrapping the leaf around the burger.

PER SERVING Calories: 150 | Fat: 5g | Protein: 23g | Sodium: 210mg | Fiber: 1g | Carbohydrates: 3g | Sugar: 1g

Red Meat Keeps Anemia at Bay

Because of your increased blood supply, your iron needs also increase during pregnancy. If you don't consume enough iron and your stores become depleted, you can become anemic. Red meat is one of the best sources of this important mineral that helps to prevent anemia.

Paleo Pumpkin Chili

This fall-inspired twist on traditional chili packs a ton of pumpkin flavor.

INGREDIENTS | SERVES 8

1 pound ground beef

1 medium yellow onion, diced

1 medium green bell pepper, diced

2 cloves garlic, minced

1 (14.5-ounce) can diced, fire-roasted tomatoes

2 (4-ounce) cans diced green chiles

1 (15-ounce) can pumpkin purée

1 cup chicken broth

1 tablespoon pumpkin pie spice

1 teaspoon chili powder

½ teaspoon sea salt

½ teaspoon black pepper

Add all ingredients to a large slow cooker and stir well. Cook on low for 7 hours until meat is cooked through. Stir well before serving to break up meat and incorporate with other ingredients.

PER SERVING Calories: 160 | Fat: 6g | Protein: 14g | Sodium: 397mg | Fiber: 3g | Carbohydrates: 13g | Sugar: 5g

Garlic Broccoli and Beef

This Asian-inspired meal is full of flavor and an unexpected ingredient—calcium. Broccoli and sesame seeds are both unexpected sources of calcium that can help you meet your daily recommendation.

INGREDIENTS | SERVES 4

¼ cup coconut aminos

1 tablespoon fresh grated ginger

2 garlic cloves, minced

½ teaspoon red pepper flakes

½ teaspoon black pepper

1 tablespoon sesame oil

1 pound beef skirt steak, thinly sliced

4 cups broccoli florets

4 medium carrots, thinly sliced

1 tablespoon sesame seeds

What Is Coconut Aminos?

Coconut aminos is a soy-free seasoning sauce made from the sap of coconut trees that tastes very similar to soy sauce. This sauce is readily available online and in most health food stores.

1. In a small bowl, whisk together coconut aminos, ginger, garlic, red pepper flakes, and black pepper. Set aside.

2. Heat sesame oil in a large wok or skillet over medium-high heat. Add steak, stirring frequently, until browned on all sides, about 5 minutes. Once the beef has browned, add in broccoli and carrots and continue to cook, stirring often.

3. Pour in coconut aminos mixture and stir well to combine. Continue to stir-fry until vegetables are softened and beef is cooked through, 2–3 minutes. Garnish with sesame seeds and serve.

PER SERVING Calories: 344 | Fat: 20g | Protein: 27g | Sodium: 675mg | Fiber: 5g | Carbohydrates: 15g | Sugar: 5g

Skillet Pork Chops and Sweet Potatoes

One-pan meals like this make cooking and cleanup a breeze. Use a cast iron skillet for perfectly seared pork chops.

INGREDIENTS | SERVES 4

4 pork chops, about ¼ pound each

Juice of 1 medium orange, divided

2 tablespoons molasses

1 tablespoon dried basil

¼ teaspoon sea salt, divided

½ teaspoon black pepper, divided

1½ tablespoons melted coconut oil, divided

1 large sweet potato, cubed

1 medium white onion, sliced

1 teaspoon cinnamon

1 teaspoon garlic powder

½ teaspoon allspice

1 tablespoon honey

1. Place pork chops in a large freezer bag with ½ of the orange juice, molasses, basil, ⅛ teaspoon salt, and ¼ teaspoon of the pepper. Shake well to evenly coat pork chops. Let marinate in the refrigerator for at least 3 hours.

2. Preheat oven to 350°F. Heat 1 tablespoon of coconut oil in a large oven-safe skillet over medium heat. While the skillet is heating, toss the sweet potatoes and onions in a large bowl with remaining orange juice and coconut oil, cinnamon, garlic, allspice, honey, and remaining salt and pepper.

3. Once skillet is hot, add sweet potatoes and onions and cook, stirring often, for 10–12 minutes, until sweet potatoes are softened. Clear space in the skillet for the pork chops by pushing the sweet potatoes and onions to the outer edge of the skillet. Place the pork chops in the middle of the skillet and sear for 2 minutes per side.

4. Add the marinating juices to the skillet and carefully transfer the skillet to the preheated oven. Roast for 20 minutes, until vegetables are tender and pork chops are cooked through.

PER SERVING Calories: 285 | Fat: 10g | Protein: 25g | Sodium: 238mg | Fiber: 2g | Carbohydrates: 24g | Sugar: 13g

Slow Cooker Pulled Pork

This simple recipe can be stored in the refrigerator or freezer and added to meals as needed. Use in a breakfast casserole, as a topping for baked sweet potatoes, or to make lunchtime lettuce wraps.

INGREDIENTS | SERVES 8

4 strips bacon
1 (3-pound) pork shoulder
½ teaspoon sea salt
1 teaspoon black pepper

Add Water As Needed

The meat should release plenty of its own juices, but if the meat doesn't have much fat and it seems a little dry as it is cooking, add ¼ to ½ cup of water to the slow cooker before shredding.

1. Lay bacon in the bottom of a large slow cooker. Place pork shoulder on top of bacon slices and wrap bacon around pork shoulder. Sprinkle evenly with salt and pepper.

2. Cook on low for 8 hours and shred with a fork before serving.

PER SERVING Calories: 377 | Fat: 25g | Protein: 36g | Sodium: 508mg | Fiber: 0g | Carbohydrates: 0g | Sugar: 0g

Steak and Pepper Fajitas

Fajitas are actually a great go-to Paleo meal—just leave out the tortillas, cheese, and sour cream. This at-home version includes all of the best parts of a restaurant-style meal. Serve with a side of salsa and Classic Guacamole (see Chapter 8).

INGREDIENTS | SERVES 4

1 tablespoon olive oil

Juice of 1 medium lime

½ teaspoon garlic powder

¼ teaspoon cumin

¼ teaspoon chili powder

½ teaspoon sea salt, divided

1 teaspoon black pepper, divided

1 pound flank steak, sliced into ½" thick strips

1 tablespoon coconut oil

3 bell peppers (1 red, 1 green, 1 yellow), stems and seeds removed, thinly sliced

1. In a small bowl, stir together olive oil, lime juice, garlic powder, cumin, chili powder, ¼ teaspoon salt, and ½ teaspoon black pepper. Place steak into a large freezer bag and pour marinade over steak. Marinate in the refrigerator for at least 3 hours or up to 24 hours.

2. Heat a large skillet or grill pan over medium-high heat. Add steak and cook for 3 minutes per side for medium-well. Discard marinade.

3. Meanwhile, in a separate large pan, heat coconut oil over medium heat. Add peppers and cook, stirring occasionally, until peppers are softened, about 5 minutes. Sprinkle with remaining salt and pepper and stir to combine.

4. Divide steak evenly between four plates and top each with fajita peppers.

PER SERVING Calories: 255 | Fat: 15g | Protein: 25g | Sodium: 360mg | Fiber: 2g | Carbohydrates: 5g | Sugar: 2g

Persian Spiced Lamb with Carrot and Fennel Slaw

The blend of Persian spices in this ground lamb dish gives it a unique and complex flavor that pairs perfectly with a fresh, crisp slaw.

INGREDIENTS | SERVES 4

4 large carrots, grated
½ cup shredded green cabbage
1 fennel bulb, thinly sliced or grated
4 celery hearts, thinly sliced
4 tablespoons olive oil
Juice of 1 large lemon
2 teaspoons coriander, divided
½ teaspoon sea salt, divided
1 teaspoon black pepper, divided
1 pound ground lamb
¼ teaspoon ground clove
¼ teaspoon cardamom
½ teaspoon garlic powder
½ teaspoon chili powder
½ teaspoon red pepper flakes
½ teaspoon turmeric
1 teaspoon cumin
1 teaspoon tarragon
1 cup snow peas
1 large handful baby spinach

1. For the slaw: Combine carrots, cabbage, fennel, and celery in a large bowl. In a small bowl, whisk together olive oil, lemon juice, 1 teaspoon coriander, ¼ teaspoon salt, and ½ teaspoon pepper. Pour dressing over slaw and stir well until vegetables are evenly coated. Store in the refrigerator until ready to use.

2. For the meat: Heat a large skillet over medium heat. While skillet is heating, place ground lamb in a large bowl with remaining salt, pepper, and other spices and mix well to incorporate. Add ground lamb to skillet and cook until browned, stirring often to break meat up as it cooks, about 8 minutes.

3. Pour in snow peas and cook until heated through, stirring occasionally, about 5 minutes. Add spinach to skillet and cook until wilted, about 3 minutes.

4. Divide slaw evenly among 4 plates and top slaw with lamb mixture.

PER SERVING Calories: 536 | Fat: 41g | Protein: 23g | Sodium: 498mg | Fiber: 8g | Carbohydrates: 21g | Sugar: 7g

Give Lamb a Try

If you've never had ground lamb, it is definitely worth a taste. The texture and flavor are similar to ground beef and it can actually be used in place of ground beef in many recipes.

Taco-less Taco Salad

This flavorful Mexican dish is bursting with spices and fresh vegetables. You won't even miss the fried corn tortilla.

INGREDIENTS | SERVES 4

1 pound ground beef

1 tablespoon chili powder

2 teaspoons paprika

1 teaspoon garlic powder

1 teaspoon cumin

1 teaspoon dried oregano

1 teaspoon sea salt, divided

1 teaspoon black pepper, divided

1 medium avocado, pitted

Juice of ½ large lime

¼ cup coconut milk

2 tablespoons water

¼ cup chopped fresh cilantro leaves

1 large head Romaine lettuce, roughly chopped

4 Roma tomatoes, sliced

½ medium red onion, diced

1 medium green bell pepper, chopped

1. In a large bowl combine ground beef, chili powder, paprika, garlic powder, cumin, oregano, ½ teaspoon salt, and ½ teaspoon pepper. Mix well to combine.

2. Heat a large skillet over medium-high heat. Add the meat and cook until fully cooked through, stirring often to break meat up as it cooks, about 8–10 minutes.

3. While meat is cooking, add avocado, lime juice, coconut milk, water, cilantro, and remaining salt and pepper to a food processor with the chopping blade attached. Process until smooth and creamy.

4. In a large salad bowl, combine lettuce, tomatoes, onion, and bell peppers. Divide the salad mixture between 4 plates, top with ground beef, and spoon avocado cream sauce on top.

PER SERVING Calories: 370 | Fat: 23g | Protein: 27g | Sodium: 707mg | Fiber: 10g | Carbohydrates: 18g | Sugar: 5g

Sun-Dried Tomato Lamb Burger

Stuffed with sun-dried tomatoes and black olives, this burger has a delicious Greek-inspired flavor in every bite!

INGREDIENTS | SERVES 4

1 pound ground lamb
¼ cup julienne-cut sun-dried tomatoes
10 black olives, sliced
½ teaspoon basil
½ teaspoon oregano
¼ teaspoon marjoram
¼ teaspoon sea salt
¼ teaspoon black pepper
1 tablespoon coconut oil

Cook Once, Eat Twice

These burgers are simple to reheat in the microwave, so they make great leftovers! Pack any extras for the next day's lunch.

1. Mix all ingredients except the coconut oil in a large bowl until well incorporated. Form mixture into 4 equal patties.

2. Heat coconut oil in a large skillet or grill pan over medium heat. Place burgers in skillet and cook, undisturbed, for 5 minutes. Flip burgers and cook for an additional 5 minutes, or to your desired level of doneness.

PER SERVING Calories: 368 | Fat: 31g | Protein: 19g | Sodium: 380mg | Fiber: 1g | Carbohydrates: 3g | Sugar: 1g

Easy Peasy Beef Roast

This tarragon-scented beef roast comes together with almost no prep work, thanks to perfectly sized peas and carrots. Throw everything together in the morning, let the slow cooker do all the work for you, and come home to a fragrant, super-nutritious dinner.

INGREDIENTS | SERVES 8

1½ teaspoons dried tarragon

1 teaspoon garlic powder

¼ teaspoon sea salt

½ teaspoon black pepper

1 (4-pound) beef chuck roast

1 cup beef stock

2 cups sugar snap peas (fresh or frozen)

1 cup baby carrots

1 medium yellow onion, cut into ½" wedges

1. In a small bowl, stir together tarragon, garlic powder, salt, and pepper. Rub spice mix evenly onto all sides of roast.

2. Pour beef stock into a large slow cooker and place the beef roast on top. Place snap peas, carrots, and onion wedges around the sides of the roast. Cook on low for 6–8 hours, until meat is tender. Slice or shred meat and serve with vegetables.

PER SERVING Calories: 419 | Fat: 21g | Protein: 46g | Sodium: 318mg | Fiber: 3g | Carbohydrates: 9g | Sugar: 4g

Sweet and Spicy Sausage Stuffed Peppers

Spicy poblanos stuffed with smoky mashed sweet potatoes and sausage—these delicious stuffed peppers are not for the faint of heart.

INGREDIENTS | SERVES 4

1 medium sweet potato, cut into large cubes

1 chipotle pepper in adobo sauce, finely chopped

4 poblano peppers

½ pound ground pork sausage

½ medium yellow onion, diced

2 cloves garlic, minced

¼ cup chopped fresh cilantro leaves

½ teaspoon paprika

½ teaspoon cumin

¼ teaspoon sea salt

½ teaspoon black pepper

1. Preheat oven to 450°F. Add 6 cups of water to a large pot over high heat. Once boiling, add sweet potatoes to pot and boil for 10 minutes, until fork tender. When potatoes are done, drain water from pot and mash sweet potatoes with chipotle pepper. Set aside.

2. While potatoes are boiling, cut tops of poblano peppers and slice in half lengthwise. Remove seeds and membrane. Place peppers on a baking sheet and roast for 15 minutes, until soft. Remove peppers from oven and let cool enough to handle.

3. Heat a large skillet over medium heat. Add sausage and brown for 3 minutes, stirring often to break up meat. Add onion and garlic to skillet and cook until softened and sausage is fully browned, about 5–7 minutes. Remove from heat and stir in cilantro, paprika, cumin, salt, and pepper.

4. Spread an even amount of sweet potato into each pepper and top with sausage mixture. Return peppers to oven for 8 minutes. Turn oven to broil and cook for an additional 2 minutes, until tops are nicely browned.

PER SERVING Calories: 231 | Fat: 15g | Protein: 10g | Sodium: 528mg | Fiber: 2g | Carbohydrates: 14g | Sugar: 5g

Grilled Pesto Steak

Pesto is a great sauce for meat as well as vegetables. Try this easy-to-cook steak topped with fresh and aromatic Paleo Pesto (see Chapter 8).

INGREDIENTS | SERVES 4

1½ pounds flank steak

2 cups Paleo Pesto, divided (see Chapter 8)

The Power of Beef

Tons of natural flavor and protein are packed into every delicious bite of organic, lean meats. You can eat more than two-thirds of your daily recommended intake for protein with just four ounces of lean beef. If you take into consideration the amount of vitamins and minerals such as B_6, B_{12}, iron, and zinc that accompany that whopping amount of protein, this small serving of meat is worth its weight in gold.

1. Place the flank steak in a large resealable plastic bag and pour 1 cup of Paleo Pesto over it. Toss to coat; marinate in the refrigerator for 4 hours.

2. Preheat a grill to medium heat, then spray or brush with oil.

3. Set steak on the grill and cook for 8–10 minutes.

4. Turn the steak, cover with remaining cup of pesto, and continue cooking for 8–10 minutes or until internal temperature reads 160°F.

5. Remove from heat, set on a platter, and tent with foil for 5–7 minutes. Slice against the grain to serve.

PER SERVING Calories: 615 | Fat: 46g | Protein: 43g | Sodium: 763mg | Fiber: 0g | Carbohydrates: 4g | Sugar: 0g

CHAPTER 10

Poultry

Basic Roasted Chicken Breasts

Use this basic chicken recipe as a jumping-off point and let your imagination take over. Add a spice rub of mixed herbs for garden-fresh flavor or heat it up with paprika and cayenne pepper.

INGREDIENTS | SERVES 4

4 boneless, skinless chicken breasts
2 tablespoons coconut oil, divided
⅛ teaspoon sea salt
⅛ teaspoon black pepper

Protein for You and Your Baby

During pregnancy, your baby is constantly growing and your own body (breasts, uterus, and placenta) is growing as well. Protein provides the building blocks to facilitate this growth, so it is important to include plenty of protein in your diet.

1. Preheat oven to 375°F. Rinse chicken and pat dry with a paper towel. Brush both sides of chicken breasts with 1 tablespoon of the coconut oil and sprinkle both sides with salt and pepper.

2. Lightly oil a large baking pan with the remaining coconut oil and place chicken breasts in pan. Roast for 25–30 minutes, until chicken is no longer pink in the middle and juices run clear.

PER SERVING Calories: 329 | Fat: 13g | Protein: 50g | Sodium: 347mg | Fiber: 0g | Carbohydrates: 0g | Sugar: 0g

Jalapeño Lime Chicken Sliders

These perfectly portioned mini burgers are great for parties (baby shower, perhaps?), or keep them all for yourself and enjoy them throughout the week. Serve them in large romaine leaves for lunch or dinner or over fluffy scrambled eggs with a side of avocado for breakfast.

INGREDIENTS | SERVES 4

1 pound ground chicken
1 jalapeño, deseeded and minced
1 tablespoon chopped fresh cilantro
1 tablespoon lime juice
1 teaspoon garlic powder
1 teaspoon paprika
⅛ teaspoon sea salt
⅛ teaspoon black pepper
1 tablespoon coconut oil

1. In a large bowl, combine chicken, jalapeño, cilantro, lime juice, garlic powder, paprika, salt, and pepper. Form into 8 small patties.

2. Heat coconut oil in a large skillet or grill pan over medium-high heat. Place burgers in skillet or grill pan and cook for 3–4 minutes per side, until chicken is no longer pink in the middle and juices run clear.

PER SERVING Calories: 272 | Fat: 21g | Protein: 20g | Sodium: 160mg | Fiber: 0g | Carbohydrates: 1g | Sugar: 0g

Baked Chicken and Peppers

This one-pan meal takes only a few minutes to prepare, giving you a chance to relax as it bakes instead of doing dishes.

INGREDIENTS | SERVES 4

2 tablespoons coconut oil, divided

2 boneless, skinless chicken breasts, cut into 1" cubes

1 large yellow onion, cut into 8 wedges

4 medium bell peppers of assorted colors, cored, seeded, and cut into ½" strips

¼ teaspoon cumin

¼ teaspoon coriander

¼ teaspoon paprika

⅛ teaspoon sea salt

⅛ teaspoon black pepper

1. Heat oven to 450°F. Coat a 13" × 9" glass baking dish with 1 tablespoon of the coconut oil.

2. Add chicken, onion, and bell peppers to baking dish. Toss with remaining oil and spices until everything is evenly coated.

3. Bake for 50–55 minutes, stirring once after 30 minutes, until chicken is cooked through and vegetables are beginning to brown.

PER SERVING Calories: 235 | Fat: 10g | Protein: 27g | Sodium: 216mg | Fiber: 3g | Carbohydrates: 9g | Sugar: 4g

Turkey-Stuffed Mushrooms

These stuffed mushrooms are overflowing with holiday flavor, thanks to fall-inspired spices and dried cherries.

INGREDIENTS | SERVES 4

4 large portobello mushrooms
2 tablespoons coconut oil, divided
½ medium white onion, diced
2 ribs celery, diced
¼ cup unsweetened dried cherries, diced
½ cup baby spinach, roughly chopped
1 clove garlic, minced
½ teaspoon dried sage
½ teaspoon dried thyme
⅛ teaspoon sea salt
⅛ teaspoon black pepper
1 pound ground turkey
1 large egg, beaten
¼ cup almond flour

1. Clean mushroom caps by gently wiping them with a damp paper towel. Remove and dice the stems and set aside. Scoop out the gills with a spoon and discard. Brush mushroom caps with 1 tablespoon of the coconut oil and place in a large glass baking dish.

2. Heat remaining coconut oil in a large skillet over medium heat. Add onions to skillet and cook until translucent, stirring often, about 3–5 minutes. Add celery, cherries, spinach, garlic, mushroom stems, and spices to skillet along with the onion. Stir well to incorporate and cook for an additional 4 minutes, stirring occasionally.

3. Add ground turkey to skillet and heat until cooked through, about 8–10 minutes, stirring occasionally to incorporate ingredients. Transfer mixture to a large bowl.

4. Stir egg and almond flour into turkey mixture until well combined.

5. Scoop an even amount of the turkey mixture into each mushroom cap. Bake for 20–25 minutes, until beginning to brown on top.

PER SERVING Calories: 321 | Fat: 21g | Protein: 25g | Sodium: 224mg | Fiber: 3g | Carbohydrates: 9g | Sugar: 5g

Turkey Roll-Ups

These roll-ups are perfectly packable when you are on the go. Serve with mustard, salsa, or Paleo Mayonnaise (see Chapter 8). To ensure the meat in this recipe is safe to eat during pregnancy, heat it until steaming and allow to cool to room temperature before eating, or you could use leftover sliced turkey breast.

INGREDIENTS | SERVES 4

8 slices organic, nitrate-free deli turkey

1 medium avocado, pitted and sliced

½ medium red bell pepper, deseeded and sliced

½ medium cucumber, cut into thin 4" long strips

Lay turkey slices out flat on a work surface. Top one half of each slice of turkey with a few slices of avocado, bell pepper, and cucumber. Tightly roll each slice of turkey around ingredients.

PER SERVING Calories: 196 | Fat: 12g | Protein: 17g | Sodium: 40mg | Fiber: 4g | Carbohydrates: 6.5g | Sugar: 1.5g

A Balanced Paleo Diet

Protein-rich turkey, avocado slices full of healthy fats, and lots of fiber and phytonutrients from the veggies make these roll-ups the very definition of a balanced Paleo meal.

Asian Chicken and Broccoli Soup

This flavorful Asian soup makes a great weeknight meal with lots of leftovers. If you make this soup at the beginning of the week, you'll have plenty left over for a busy night or two.

INGREDIENTS | SERVES 8

6 cups chicken stock

6 boneless, skinless chicken thighs

1 large yellow onion, chopped

10–12 button mushrooms, sliced

2 garlic cloves, thinly sliced

1 large bunch broccoli, stems removed, chopped into florets

1 tablespoon coconut aminos

1 teaspoon red chili flakes

1 teaspoon ground ginger

⅛ teaspoon sea salt

⅛ teaspoon black pepper

1. Add all ingredients to slow cooker and stir well to combine. Cook on low for 6–8 hours.

2. Shred chicken with a fork before serving.

PER SERVING Calories: 150 | Fat: 4g | Protein: 16.5g | Sodium: 415mg | Fiber: 1g | Carbohydrates: 11g | Sugar: 4.5g

Slow Cooker Thanksgiving Turkey Breast

Perfectly spiced turkey among fall vegetables and fresh cranberries—it's all the flavor of Thanksgiving dinner, without all the work!

INGREDIENTS | SERVES 6

1 tablespoon orange zest
1 teaspoon dried thyme
½ teaspoon dried rosemary
½ teaspoon dried basil
½ teaspoon dried sage
⅛ teaspoon sea salt
⅛ teaspoon black pepper
1 (2½–3 pound) boneless turkey breast
1 large white onion, sliced
1 cup baby carrots
1 medium sweet potato, peeled and cut into 1½" cubes
1 cup fresh cranberries
2 tablespoons orange juice
½ cup water

1. In a small bowl, stir together orange zest, thyme, rosemary, basil, sage, salt, and pepper. Rub turkey breast on all sides with spice mix and place in bottom of slow cooker.

2. Arrange onion, carrots, and sweet potato around turkey. Scatter cranberries on top. Pour orange juice and water evenly into slow cooker.

3. Cook on low for 5–6 hours, until turkey is cooked through and vegetables are soft.

PER SERVING Calories: 297 | Fat: 1.5g | Protein: 56g | Sodium: 185mg | Fiber: 2.5g | Carbohydrates: 11g | Sugar: 4g

Hawaiian Turkey Burgers

Burgers are so much fun because there are so many flavor and topping combinations. These island-flavored burgers are served over a simple slaw and topped with fresh, juicy pineapple.

INGREDIENTS | SERVES 4

1 pound ground turkey
¼ teaspoon sea salt, divided
¼ teaspoon black pepper, divided
2 green onions, diced
1 tablespoon coconut aminos
1 teaspoon hot sauce
1 tablespoon coconut oil
2 cups shredded red cabbage
1 teaspoon olive oil
Juice of ½ large lime
4 fresh pineapple rings

Easy Pineapple Slices

Did you know you can buy an inexpensive pineapple slicer that will quickly core and slice a pineapple into perfect rings? Most major retailers carry these products or you can search online for "pineapple slicer."

1. In a large bowl, combine ground turkey, ⅛ teaspoon salt, ⅛ teaspoon pepper, green onions, coconut aminos, and hot sauce. Mix well to combine, and form into 4 equal patties.

2. Heat coconut oil in a large skillet or grill pan over medium heat. Place burgers in skillet and cook, undisturbed, for 5 minutes. Flip burgers and cook for an additional 5 minutes, or to your desired level of doneness.

3. While burgers are cooking, stir together cabbage, olive oil, lime juice, and remaining salt and pepper in a medium bowl. Divide slaw evenly among 4 plates.

4. Place burgers over slaw and top each with a slice of pineapple.

PER SERVING Calories: 305 | Fat: 14g | Protein: 21g | Sodium: 429mg | Fiber: 3g | Carbohydrates: 25g | Sugar: 18g

Farmers' Market Chicken Bake

This chicken bake tastes rich and feels indulgent, but it is chock full of healthy ingredients! Roasting the butternut squash and apples provides a sweetness that pairs well with the herb-infused chicken and crispy, salty bacon.

INGREDIENTS | SERVES 4

2 tablespoons coconut oil, divided

2 boneless skinless chicken breasts, cut into 1" cubes

1 Golden Delicious apple, cut into 1" cubes

1 large yellow onion, cut into 8 wedges

1 small butternut squash, peeled, deseeded, and cut into 1" cubes

½ teaspoon cardamom

1 teaspoon chopped fresh thyme

1 tablespoon chopped fresh sage

1 teaspoon chopped fresh rosemary

⅛ teaspoon sea salt

⅛ teaspoon black pepper

6 slices bacon

1. Heat oven to 450°F. Coat a 13" × 9" glass baking dish with 1 tablespoon of coconut oil.

2. Add chicken, apple, onion, and squash to baking dish. Toss with remaining coconut oil and spices until everything is evenly coated.

3. Lay bacon slices evenly across the top of the dish. Bake for 50–55 minutes, until bacon is crispy, chicken is cooked through, and vegetables are beginning to brown.

PER SERVING Calories: 429 | Fat: 25g | Protein: 31g | Sodium: 500mg | Fiber: 3g | Carbohydrates: 21g | Sugar: 8g

Turkey and Veggie Meatloaf

Meatloaf is an American classic, but this version is lightened up with fresh vegetables and mild ground turkey.

A Perfect "First Food" for Baby

Once your baby is eating finger foods, this meatloaf would be a wonderful dinner to share with him. Even if he only has a few teeth, he will enjoy the tender ground turkey and soft vegetables. If your baby is sensitive to or not a fan of spicy foods, feel free to omit the black pepper, paprika, and/or chili powder from this recipe.

1. Heat oven to 375°F. Grease a loaf pan with the coconut oil.

2. Combine turkey, egg, 2 tablespoons tomato paste, onion, carrots, zucchini, spinach, 1 teaspoon garlic powder, paprika, ⅛ teaspoon salt, and ⅛ teaspoon pepper in a large bowl. Mix well to combine.

3. Spread turkey mixture evenly into loaf pan. Bake for 50 minutes.

4. While meatloaf is baking, combine ½ cup tomato paste, water, apple cider vinegar, ½ teaspoon garlic powder, chili powder, and remaining salt and pepper in a small saucepan over medium-low heat. Simmer for 10 minutes, stirring often.

5. After 50 minutes, remove meatloaf from oven and drain any excess liquid from the loaf pan. Spread sauce evenly over top of the meatloaf. Return to the oven and cook for an additional 10 minutes.

PER SERVING Calories: 210 | Fat: 11g | Protein: 22g | Sodium: 360mg | Fiber: 1.5g | Carbohydrates: 6g | Sugar: 3g

Spice-Rubbed Roasted Turkey Breast

Turkey breast is protein-packed and can be made as flavorful as you want. This spice-rubbed recipe combines an abundance of tasty spices that infuse the turkey breast with delicious flavor.

INGREDIENTS | SERVES 8

2 tablespoons coconut oil, divided

1 (5-pound) turkey breast, thawed

2 teaspoons garlic powder

2 teaspoons onion powder

1 teaspoon cayenne

1 teaspoon sea salt

1 teaspoon black pepper

1 medium lemon, sliced

1. Preheat oven to 325°F, and grease a roasting pan with 1 tablespoon of coconut oil. Set the turkey breast in roasting pan (make sure it is thawed).

2. Combine the garlic powder, onion powder, cayenne, sea salt, and pepper in a small mixing bowl and mix well.

3. Coat the turkey breast with the remaining coconut oil, and sprinkle spice mixture over the turkey breast. Top with lemon slices.

4. Cook the turkey breast for 1½–2½ hours, or until internal temperature reads 165–170°F.

PER SERVING Calories: 331 | Fat: 4g | Protein: 69g | Sodium: 433mg | Fiber: 0.28g | Carbohydrates: 2g | Sugar: 0.08g

Lemon-Basil Chicken

Plain chicken breasts get a complete makeover with this recipe. Spices and fresh lemon make this dish flavorful, juicy, and moist.

INGREDIENTS | SERVES 2

2 boneless, skinless chicken breasts

Juice from 1 medium lemon

1 teaspoon sea salt

1 teaspoon garlic powder

2 teaspoons Italian seasoning

4 tablespoons chopped fresh basil leaves

1 medium lemon, sliced

Chicken for Versatile, Clean Protein

Brimming with protein and important B vitamins, chicken can be prepared in an astounding number of ways—so don't let it get boring! Whether it's grilled, broiled, blackened, roasted, sautéed, or baked, you can dress up this lean meat with spices and sauces, and serve it with vegetables or even fruit. The possibilities are endless, and the health benefits are perfect for you and your growing baby.

1. Preheat oven to 350°F, and grease a 9" × 9" casserole dish with oil.

2. Place chicken breasts in the casserole dish and pour lemon juice over them.

3. Sprinkle the breasts with salt, garlic powder, Italian seasoning, and basil leaves.

4. Cover the seasoned breasts with the lemon slices, and cook for 20–25 minutes, or until cooked thoroughly and juices run clear.

PER SERVING Calories: 156 | Fat: 4g | Protein: 25g | Sodium: 1,267mg | Fiber: 2g | Carbohydrates: 7g | Sugar: 1.5g

Citrus Chicken Kebabs

Delectable citrus fruit gets skewered between juicy pieces of chicken breast in this recipe, creating a unique flavor combination you're sure to enjoy. Packed with abundant nutrition, this meal is a great alternative to traditional chicken recipes.

INGREDIENTS | SERVES 2

2 boneless, skinless chicken breasts
2 large grapefruits
1 pineapple

1. Cut chicken breasts into ½" thick squares.

2. Remove the grapefruit rind, separate the sections, and cut them into ¼" pieces. Remove the top and outside of the pineapple, and cut into ¼" squares.

3. Preheat a grill to medium heat, then spray or brush with oil.

4. On four skewers, stack the chicken, pineapple, and grapefruit pieces (in that order) until all ingredients are skewered. Lay skewers on hot grill surface.

5. Turn frequently, and remove when chicken is completely cooked through or after about 10 minutes.

PER SERVING Calories: 308 | Fat: 0.80g | Protein: 4g | Sodium: 5mg | Fiber: 9g | Carbohydrates: 80g | Sugar: 63g

Fish and Seafood

Salmon Muffins

Easy to prepare, and easy to freeze, these salmon muffins are a perfect pregnancy food. Whip up a double batch and freeze in an airtight container for a quick protein-rich meal when you just don't have time to cook.

INGREDIENTS | SERVES 4

1 tablespoon coconut oil

16 ounces canned salmon (preferably canned with skin and bones)

1 rib celery, roughly chopped

½ medium yellow onion, roughly chopped

1 large egg

¼ cup julienne-cut sun-dried tomatoes

1 teaspoon garlic powder

1 tablespoon chopped fresh flat-leaf parsley

⅛ teaspoon sea salt

⅛ teaspoon black pepper

1. Preheat oven to 350°F. Grease a muffin tin with coconut oil (or use a silicon muffin pan).

2. Add remaining ingredients to food processor and process until well combined. Scoop about ¼ cup of the salmon mixture into each muffin tin.

3. Bake for 30–35 minutes, until the muffins are cooked through and just beginning to brown around the edges.

PER SERVING Calories: 253 | Fat: 13g | Protein: 28g | Sodium: 575mg | Fiber: 1g | Carbohydrates: 4g | Sugar: 2g

Skin and Bones

When you purchase salmon that is canned with the skin and bones, you get even more omega-3 fats and healthy doses of calcium and vitamin D. When the salmon is mixed in a food processor, such as with this recipe, you probably won't even notice these extras.

Lemon Pepper Shrimp Skewers

These skewers are a great choice for lightened-up grilling fare. Taking a little extra time to let the shrimp marinate really allows them to soak up the bright, lemony flavor.

INGREDIENTS | SERVES 4

1 pound medium or medium–large shrimp, peeled and deveined

Juice of 2 medium lemons

1 tablespoon ghee, melted

½ teaspoon garlic powder

⅛ teaspoon sea salt

1 teaspoon black pepper

1. Combine shrimp and lemon juice in a large resealable bag. Marinate in the refrigerator for at least 30 minutes or up to 3 hours.

2. Thread shrimp onto 4 skewers. Brush shrimp with melted ghee and sprinkle with garlic powder, salt, and pepper. Flip skewers and repeat on second side.

3. Heat a grill or grill pan over medium heat. Place skewers on grill for 4–5 minutes on each side, until shrimp turns pink and is just cooked through.

PER SERVING Calories: 152 | Fat: 5g | Protein: 23g | Sodium: 242mg | Fiber: 0g | Carbohydrates: 2g | Sugar: 0g

Lime Grilled Ahi Tuna with Pineapple Slaw

Tuna is a rich and meaty fish, so the rest of this dish is kept light with a sweet and tangy pineapple slaw.

INGREDIENTS | SERVES 4

2 ahi tuna steaks, about ½ pound each

1 tablespoon coconut oil, melted

¼ teaspoon sea salt, divided

¼ teaspoon pepper, divided

Juice of 2 medium limes, divided

3 cups shredded purple cabbage

1 cup chopped pineapple

1 cup grated carrots

1 tablespoon olive oil

2 tablespoons apple cider vinegar

Avoiding Undercooked Fish During Pregnancy

Ahi tuna steaks are typically served rare, but during pregnancy it is important to thoroughly heat seafood before eating to avoid foodborne illnesses.

1. Heat a grill over medium-high heat. Pat tuna steaks dry with a paper towel and set on a plate or cutting board. Brush with coconut oil and sprinkle with ⅛ teaspoon salt and ⅛ teaspoon pepper on both sides.

2. Place steaks on grill and cook with lid closed for 4–5 minutes per side, until no longer pink in the center. Squeeze juice of 1 lime over steaks and remove from grill to rest while you prepare the slaw.

3. In a large bowl, stir together cabbage, pineapple, carrots, olive oil, vinegar, juice of 1 lime, and remaining salt and pepper. Divide slaw evenly among 4 plates. Serve with tuna steaks.

PER SERVING Calories: 270 | Fat: 12g | Protein: 27g | Sodium: 222mg | Fiber: 3g | Carbohydrates: 12g | Sugar: 7g

Cedar Plank Salmon with Grilled Peaches

Because it takes a little extra time and preparation, this meal is perfect for weekend grilling with friends and family. Serve with a side of string beans to get your greens in!

INGREDIENTS | SERVES 4

2 cedar grill planks

2 salmon filets, about ½ pound each

1 tablespoon melted coconut oil, divided

2 teaspoons honey, divided

Juice of 1 medium lime, divided

¼ teaspoon sea salt, divided

⅛ teaspoon black pepper

½ teaspoon chili powder

½ teaspoon garlic powder

2 large peaches

1. Fully submerge planks in water and soak for 1 hour. While planks are soaking, prepare your salmon and peaches.

2. Place salmon on a plate, skin side down. In a small bowl, combine ½ tablespoon of coconut oil, 1 teaspoon of honey, juice of ½ lime, ⅛ teaspoon of salt, pepper, chili powder, and garlic powder. Brush mixture onto skinless side of salmon filets.

3. Cut peaches in half and remove pits. Place on a plate, cut side up. Sprinkle with remaining salt and drizzle with remaining coconut oil and honey.

4. Preheat grill to medium heat. Add soaked planks to grill rack. Cover and heat for 3 minutes. Flip planks over and place salmon, skin side down, on one plank and peaches, cut side down, on the other. Close grill lid and cook for 15 minutes, undisturbed.

5. Open grill and squeeze remaining lime juice onto salmon. Close grill lid and continue to cook until salmon flakes easily, about 10–15 minutes more.

PER SERVING Calories: 231 | Fat: 11g | Protein: 23g | Sodium: 200mg | Fiber: 1g | Carbohydrates: 11g | Sugar: 9g

Broiled Tilapia with Pistachio Cherry Sauce

The sweetness of the cherry sauce balances out the heat from the chipotle peppers in this tasty seafood dish.

INGREDIENTS | SERVES 4

1 tablespoon melted ghee, divided
4 (6-ounce) tilapia filets
⅛ teaspoon sea salt
⅛ teaspoon black pepper
¼ teaspoon ground chipotle pepper
1 cup frozen cherries
Juice of 1 large lemon
½ teaspoon cinnamon
½ cup raw shelled pistachios

Spicy Foods and Heartburn

People who suffer from heartburn, a common pregnancy symptom, are often advised to avoid spicy foods. If you are experiencing heartburn regularly, try omitting hot peppers and spices from recipes to see if you can find some relief.

1. Preheat oven to broil. Brush a small baking dish with ½ tablespoon of the ghee.

2. Place tilapia filets in baking dish in a single layer. Brush remaining ghee over filets and season with salt, pepper, and chipotle pepper. Broil until cooked through and flakes easily, 6–8 minutes.

3. For the sauce: in a small saucepan over low heat, combine cherries, lemon juice, and cinnamon. Cook for 15 minutes, stirring occasionally, until cherries begin to break down and sauce thickens. Stir in pistachios. Spoon evenly over filets and serve.

PER SERVING Calories: 272 | Fat: 11g | Protein: 33g | Sodium: 166mg | Fiber: 2g | Carbohydrates: 9g | Sugar: 5g

Garlic Rainbow Chard with Butternut Squash and Salmon

A hearty, warming meal for a cool winter night.
This dish proves that comfort food can be healthy, too.

INGREDIENTS | SERVES 4

1 medium butternut squash, peeled, seeded, and cut into 1" cubes

3 tablespoons ghee, divided

¼ teaspoon sea salt, divided

¼ teaspoon black pepper, divided

1 bunch of rainbow Swiss chard

4 cloves garlic, thinly sliced

½ teaspoon red chili flakes

Juice of ½ medium lemon

12 ounces canned salmon (preferably canned with skin and bones)

1. Preheat oven to 400°F. In a large glass baking dish, toss butternut squash cubes with 1 tablespoon of ghee, ⅛ teaspoon salt, and ⅛ teaspoon pepper. Roast for 25 minutes, stirring once after 10 minutes. After stirring, start preparing your other ingredients.

2. Roughly chop chard stems and set aside. Roughly chop leaves into 1" strips.

3. Heat 1 tablespoon ghee in a large skillet over medium-high heat. Add garlic and chili flakes to pan and cook, stirring frequently, until fragrant, about 3 minutes. Add chard stems to pan. Stir to incorporate with garlic. Cover and cook for 2 minutes.

4. Add remaining ghee to pan. Once melted, add chard leaves, lemon juice, and remaining salt and pepper. Stir well and cover. Cook for 3–5 minutes, until chard is wilted, but still bright.

5. Remove from heat; stir in salmon and roasted squash. Cover to keep warm until ready to serve.

PER SERVING Calories: 282 | Fat: 16g | Protein: 21g | Sodium: 513mg | Fiber: 2.5g | Carbohydrates: 14.5g | Sugar: 3g

Curried Mahi Mahi

Mahi mahi is a light, mild fish that really takes on the flavor of the curry in this meal. Spice it up with a bit of cayenne pepper if you like heat.

INGREDIENTS | SERVES 4

1 pound mahi mahi filets, cut into 1" cubes

2 tablespoons curry powder, divided

1 teaspoon cayenne pepper (optional)

2 tablespoons coconut oil

1 small white onion, sliced

1 medium red bell pepper, sliced

1 medium green bell pepper, sliced

½ cup shredded cabbage

⅛ teaspoon sea salt

⅛ teaspoon black pepper

1 small avocado, peeled, pitted, and sliced

What Is in Curry Powder Anyway?

Traditionally used in South Asian cuisine, most curry spice blends contain coriander, cumin, fennel, turmeric, fenugreek, and ground red pepper.

1. Place mahi mahi cubes in a large freezer bag. Sprinkle 1 tablespoon curry powder and cayenne pepper (optional) in bag. Shake well to evenly coat fish with spices.

2. Heat coconut oil in a large skillet over medium heat. Add onions and cook until translucent, stirring often, 2–3 minutes. Add peppers and cabbage to skillet and cook for an additional 3 minutes, stirring often.

3. Add mahi mahi, salt, pepper, and remaining tablespoon of curry powder to skillet and stir well to mix curry with vegetables. Cook for 10–12 minutes, until fish is white and flaky and vegetables are softened. Serve with a side of sliced avocado.

PER SERVING Calories: 270 | Fat: 15.5g | Protein: 23g | Sodium: 182mg | Fiber: 6g | Carbohydrates: 11g | Sugar: 3g

Summer Vegetable Haddock Bake

This summery dish incorporates garden-fresh vegetables with herb-infused haddock filets. Cooking it all in a foil-lined pan makes cleanup a cinch.

INGREDIENTS | SERVES 4

2 medium zucchini, sliced into ¼" thick slices

1 medium yellow crookneck squash, sliced into ¼" slices

12 cherry tomatoes, stems removed and halved

2 garlic cloves, minced

2 tablespoons coconut oil, divided

Juice of 1 large lemon, divided

1½ tablespoons dried dill, divided

¼ teaspoon sea salt, divided

¼ teaspoon black pepper, divided

4 haddock filets, about ¼ pound each

8 sprigs fresh thyme

12 kalamata olives, sliced

2 tablespoons capers

1. Preheat oven to 425°F.

2. Place zucchini, crookneck squash, and tomatoes into a large bowl with minced garlic. Drizzle with 1 tablespoon of the coconut oil and ½ of the lemon juice. Season with 1 tablespoon dill, ⅛ teaspoon of the salt, and ⅛ teaspoon of the pepper. Stir well to evenly coat vegetables.

3. Line a 9" × 13" glass baking dish with foil. Place haddock filets in dish. Drizzle remaining coconut oil and lemon juice over fish filets. Season with remaining salt, pepper, and dill. Pour vegetables into the pan, evenly covering the fish filets. Place thyme sprigs on top of vegetables.

4. Cover baking dish with foil and roast for 25 minutes. Remove foil from pan. Remove thyme sprigs and sprinkle olives and capers evenly over vegetables. Return to oven and cook, uncovered, for an additional 5–10 minutes, until fish is white and flaky and vegetables are soft.

PER SERVING Calories: 290 | Fat: 15g | Protein: 24g | Sodium: 368mg | Fiber: 3g | Carbohydrates: 16.5g | Sugar: 5.5g

Sweet and Spicy Fish Tacos

This dish puts a tropical twist on fish tacos with a mango salsa, while butter lettuce leaves stand in for traditional corn tortillas.

INGREDIENTS | SERVES 4

2 teaspoons melted ghee, divided

Juice of 1 medium lime, divided

1 teaspoon paprika

¼ teaspoon cayenne pepper

¼ teaspoon sea salt, divided

¼ teaspoon black pepper, divided

4 (6-ounce) tilapia filets, cut into 1" cubes

1 large mango, peeled, pitted, and cut into 1" cubes

1 medium red bell pepper, diced

1 medium avocado, peeled, pitted, and diced

12 butter lettuce leaves

1. In a small bowl, whisk together 1 teaspoon ghee, ½ of the lime juice, paprika, cayenne pepper, ⅛ teaspoon salt, and ⅛ teaspoon pepper. Brush mixture over fish filets.

2. Heat remaining ghee in a large skillet over medium heat. Place fish in skillet and cook, undisturbed, for 4 minutes. Flip and cook for an additional 3–4 minutes until fish is white and flaky.

3. While fish is cooking, stir together mango, bell pepper, and avocado with remaining lime juice, salt, and pepper in a medium bowl and set aside.

4. When fish is cooked, fill each butter lettuce leaf with the mango salsa mixture and top with fish pieces.

PER SERVING Calories: 294 | Fat: 11g | Protein: 32.5g | Sodium: 265mg | Fiber: 6g | Carbohydrates: 17.5g | Sugar: 10g

CHAPTER 12

Healthy Sides

Baked Sweet Potato Fries

Baked sweet potato fries are much healthier than the deep-fried versions you'll find at most restaurants. Don't crowd these fries in the pan—give them plenty of room to cook so they crisp up.

INGREDIENTS | SERVES 4

2 large sweet potatoes
2 tablespoons ghee
⅛ teaspoon sea salt
¼ teaspoon black pepper

Sweet-er Potatoes

To make these sweet potatoes an even sweeter treat, add ½ teaspoon of cinnamon and ¼ teaspoon of nutmeg to the spice mix.

1. Preheat oven to 450°F.

2. Scrub and rinse potatoes and dry well. Cut potatoes in half lengthwise. Cut each half lengthwise into 3 or 4 slices. Cut each slice into thin sticks, about ½" thick.

3. In a large bowl, toss potatoes with ghee, salt, and pepper. Place fries on a large foil-lined baking sheet in an even layer so they aren't touching (use two baking sheets if necessary).

4. Bake for 15 minutes. Remove from oven and flip fries using tongs or a spatula. Return to oven and bake for an additional 10 minutes, until soft in the middle and beginning to brown and crisp on the outside.

PER SERVING Calories: 112 | Fat: 6g | Protein: 1g | Sodium: 110mg | Fiber: 2g | Carbohydrates: 13g | Sugar: 3g

Harvest Brussels Sprouts

Brussels sprouts and apples go together like . . . peas and carrots. This sweet and nutty dish is packed with vitamins and minerals and makes enough to feed a crowd.

INGREDIENTS | SERVES 8

2 tablespoons ghee

2 pounds Brussels sprouts, trimmed and quartered

2 medium yellow onions, diced

2 medium Gala apples, cut into 1" cubes

2 tablespoons balsamic vinegar

1 teaspoon dried sage

1 teaspoon dried rosemary

⅛ teaspoon sea salt

⅛ teaspoon black pepper

¼ cup chopped walnuts

What's in a Name?

When you hear "dark leafy greens" you may only think of spinach, collard greens, and kale, but this family also includes vegetables such as broccoli, cabbage, and Brussels sprouts. All are good sources of prenatal nutrients, including magnesium, calcium, vitamin A, the B vitamins, vitamin C, and vitamin K.

1. Preheat oven to 400°F.

2. In a large bowl, add ghee, Brussels sprouts, onions, apples, vinegar, sage, rosemary, salt, and pepper to a large bowl and stir well to evenly coat everything with ghee and spices. Pour mixture into a 9" × 13" glass baking dish. Bake for 25 minutes.

3. After 25 minutes, remove Brussels sprouts from oven. Add walnuts to baking dish and stir well to incorporate. Return to oven for an additional 15–20 minutes, until apples are softened and Brussels sprouts are beginning to brown.

PER SERVING Calories: 135 | Fat: 6g | Protein: 5g | Sodium: 67mg | Fiber: 5.5g | Carbohydrates: 19g | Sugar: 8g

Cauliflower Rice

Use this rice as a base to make non-Paleo meals into Paleo meals. Serve it with curry, jambalaya, or chicken stir-fry.

INGREDIENTS | SERVES 4

1 large head cauliflower
2 tablespoons ghee
⅛ teaspoon sea salt
¼ teaspoon black pepper

Quick Trick: Veggie Fried Rice

Turn this basic cauliflower rice into veggie fried rice by sautéing ½ finely diced red bell pepper, ½ cup frozen snow peas, and 1 diced carrot in pan for 5 minutes before adding cauliflower.

1. Remove leaves and core from cauliflower. Chop the cauliflower into small florets. In batches, place florets into food processor with the chopping blade attached. Process until finely chopped, similar to the consistency of rice.

2. Heat ghee in a large pan over medium heat. Once melted, add cauliflower to pan and stir to coat with the ghee. Season with salt and pepper. Cover and cook for 5–7 minutes, until cauliflower is softened.

PER SERVING Calories: 92 | Fat: 7g | Protein: 3g | Sodium: 117mg | Fiber: 3g | Carbohydrates: 7g | Sugar: 2.5g

Spicy Grilled Asparagus

Many people find asparagus bland, but this recipe brightens this green veggie up with a burst of lemon, while the crushed red pepper adds a little kick.

INGREDIENTS | SERVES 4

1 pound asparagus spears, tough white ends trimmed

2 tablespoons melted ghee

Juice of ½ large lemon

1 tablespoon crushed red pepper

¼ teaspoon sea salt

¼ teaspoon black pepper

1. In a large bowl, toss asparagus spears with ghee, lemon juice, crushed red pepper, salt, and pepper.

2. Preheat large cast iron skillet or grill pan over medium-high heat. Grill for 8–10 minutes, using tongs to turn every couple of minutes, until crisp-tender and beginning to brown.

PER SERVING Calories: 84 | Fat: 6.5g | Protein: 3g | Sodium: 150mg | Fiber: 3g | Carbohydrates: 5g | Sugar: 2g

Bell Pepper and Onion Hash

This vegetarian hash can be topped with a fried egg for a quick meal.

INGREDIENTS | SERVES 4

1 tablespoon ghee

1 large red bell pepper, deseeded and diced

1 large green bell pepper, deseeded and diced

1 medium yellow onion, diced

¼ teaspoon sea salt

¼ teaspoon black pepper

1. Heat ghee in a large skillet over medium heat.

2. Add bell peppers, onion, salt, and black pepper. Cook, stirring occasionally, until vegetables are soft and golden, 8–10 minutes.

PER SERVING Calories: 55 | Fat: 3g | Protein: 1g | Sodium: 151mg | Fiber: 1.5g | Carbohydrates: 6g | Sugar: 3g

Roasted Squash

Roasting brings out the rich flavors of these squashes, giving this healthy dish an indulgent feel.

INGREDIENTS | SERVES 4

2 medium zucchini, cut into ½" thick slices

2 medium yellow squash, cut into ½" thick slices

2 tablespoons coconut oil

½ teaspoon dried basil

½ teaspoon dried oregano

⅛ teaspoon sea salt

⅛ teaspoon black pepper

Why Sea Salt?

Sea salt and other natural salts are higher in minerals—including calcium, potassium, magnesium, sulfur, zinc, and iron—than refined salts. When salt is chemically processed, the minerals are removed and various additives often take their place. Look for salt labeled "unrefined" to make sure you are getting all of the health benefits salt has to offer.

1. Preheat oven to 425°F.

2. In a large bowl, toss zucchini and yellow squash with coconut oil, basil, oregano, sea salt, and black pepper until vegetables are evenly coated. Arrange in an even layer on a large rimmed baking sheet (use two sheets if necessary so vegetables are not overcrowded).

3. Roast for 20–25 minutes until vegetables are tender and golden, stirring halfway through.

PER SERVING Calories: 96 | Fat: 7g | Protein: 2g | Sodium: 84mg | Fiber: 2g | Carbohydrates: 7g | Sugar: 6g

Mediterranean Green Beans with Golden Raisins

You won't have to force anyone to eat their vegetables with this dish. Accompanied by salty bacon, sweet golden raisins, crunchy pistachios, and fresh herbs, these green beans will have even veggie-phobes asking for seconds.

INGREDIENTS | SERVES 8

4 cups green beans, trimmed

4 slices bacon

2 garlic cloves, minced

½ large white onion, thinly sliced

¼ cup shelled pistachios

¼ cup golden raisins

1 teaspoon chopped fresh oregano

½ teaspoon chopped fresh dill

Juice of ½ medium lemon

⅛ teaspoon sea salt

¼ teaspoon black pepper

Choosing the Best Bacon

All bacon is not created equal! Look for "nitrate-free" and "uncured" on the label. Flip the package over and check out the ingredients for other additives and preservatives, as well.

1. Bring a large pot of water to a boil over high heat. When water begins to boil, add beans and simmer for 3–4 minutes, until tender. Drain water from pot and set beans aside.

2. Add bacon to a large cold skillet and heat over medium heat. Cook until evenly browned and beginning to crisp, flipping often, for about 5 minutes. Remove to a paper towel–lined plate and set aside.

3. In the same skillet, add garlic, onion, and green beans to the bacon fat and continue to cook over medium heat, stirring occasionally, for 6–8 minutes until beans are just beginning to brown.

4. When bacon has cooled enough to handle, crumble the bacon and add it to the pan along with the pistachios, golden raisins, oregano, and dill. Stir well and cook for an additional 2 minutes. Season with lemon juice, salt, and pepper.

PER SERVING Calories: 109 | Fat: 7g | Protein: 3g | Sodium: 136mg | Fiber: 2g | Carbohydrates: 10g | Sugar: 5g

Garlic-Roasted Broccoli

This roasted broccoli is easy to make and can be served with pretty much any main dish. Pair it with steak and a baked sweet potato for a decadent dinner.

INGREDIENTS | SERVES 4

1 large head broccoli, cut into florets
2 tablespoons melted ghee
3 cloves of garlic, sliced
⅛ teaspoon sea salt
½ teaspoon black pepper
½ teaspoon red pepper flakes (optional)

1. Preheat oven to 425°F.

2. In a large bowl, toss the broccoli florets with the ghee, garlic, salt, pepper, and red pepper flakes (optional).

3. Spread the broccoli in an even layer on a large baking sheet. Roast for 20 minutes until broccoli is just beginning to brown and crisp around the edges, stirring halfway through.

PER SERVING Calories: 112 | Fat: 7g | Protein: 4.5g | Sodium: 124mg | Fiber: 4g | Carbohydrates: 11g | Sugar: 2.5g

Cinnamon Skillet Carrots

These colorful, skillet-roasted carrots have a sweet and smoky taste and will look beautiful on your plate.

INGREDIENTS | SERVES 4

1 pound slender multicolored carrots, peeled

2 tablespoons melted ghee, divided

½ teaspoon cinnamon

¼ teaspoon ground ginger

¼ teaspoon ground nutmeg

⅛ teaspoon sea salt

⅛ teaspoon black pepper

A Carrot of a Different Color

Though orange carrots are the most common variety, carrots actually come in a rainbow of colors from yellow to purple—even red. Each contains different phytonutrients, which provide their various hues. Eating a rainbow of carrots means you'll also be getting a wide range of health-protective benefits.

1. In a large bowl, toss carrots with 1 tablespoon ghee, cinnamon, ginger, nutmeg, salt, and pepper.

2. Heat remaining tablespoon melted ghee in a large cast iron skillet over medium-high heat. Once hot, add the carrots to the pan in a single layer and cook, turning occasionally until all sides are browned and carrots are soft, about 12–15 minutes.

PER SERVING Calories: 104 | Fat: 6.5g | Protein: 1g | Sodium: 151mg | Fiber: 3g | Carbohydrates: 11g | Sugar: 5g

CHAPTER 13

Salads and Dressings

California Salad

This light, summery salad combines fresh strawberries and creamy avocado with a homemade balsamic dressing.

INGREDIENTS | SERVES 4

4 slices bacon

4 cups mixed lettuce greens

12 medium strawberries, sliced

4 green onions, thinly sliced

½ cup shelled pistachios

1 medium avocado, pitted and sliced

4 tablespoons Basic Vinaigrette (see recipe in this chapter)

1. Add bacon to a large cold skillet and heat over medium heat. Cook until evenly browned and just beginning to crisp, flipping often, for about 5 minutes. Remove to a paper towel–lined plate and set aside.

2. In a large bowl, toss together mixed greens, strawberries, green onions, and pistachios. Once bacon has cooled, crumble and sprinkle over salad.

3. Divide salad evenly between 4 bowls. Top each salad with avocado slices and drizzle each with 1 tablespoon Basic Vinaigrette.

PER SERVING Calories: 362 | Fat: 32g | Protein: 7.5g | Sodium: 204mg | Fiber: 6g | Carbohydrates: 13g | Sugar: 4.5g

Paleo Cobb Salad

A Paleo take on the traditional Cobb salad. Canned chicken makes for an easy shortcut, but you can also use chopped leftover chicken breasts.

INGREDIENTS | SERVES 4

4 slices bacon

4 cups chopped romaine lettuce

1 (12.5-ounce) can chunk chicken breast, drained (no additives or preservatives)

1 cup cherry tomatoes, halved

½ small red onion, diced

1 medium avocado, pitted and sliced

2 large hard-boiled eggs, sliced

4 tablespoons Basic Vinaigrette (see recipe in this chapter)

The Perfect Food

Have you ever heard eggs referred to as "nature's perfect food"? Eggs are packed with protein, as well as saturated and unsaturated fats. They also contain a variety of vitamins, minerals, and antioxidants, especially in the yolks.

1. Add bacon to a large cold skillet and heat over medium heat. Cook until evenly browned and just beginning to crisp, flipping often, for about 5 minutes. Remove to a paper towel–lined plate and set aside.

2. In a large bowl, toss together chopped romaine, chicken breast, tomatoes, and red onion. Once bacon has cooled, crumble and sprinkle over salad.

3. Divide salad evenly between 4 bowls. Top each salad with avocado and egg slices and drizzle each with 1 tablespoon Basic Vinaigrette.

PER SERVING Calories: 352 | Fat: 31g | Protein: 7g | Sodium: 197mg | Fiber: 6g | Carbohydrates: 13g | Sugar: 5g

Salmon and Citrus Salad

This "no-cook" salad is easy enough to pack for lunch and tasty enough to serve to a crowd.

INGREDIENTS | SERVES 4

4 cups spring mix greens

8 mandarin oranges, peeled and segmented

½ medium cucumber, thinly sliced

½ small red onion, thinly sliced

10 ounces canned salmon, drained

4 tablespoons Avocado Cream Sauce (see recipe in this chapter)

1. Toss spring mix, oranges, cucumber, red onion, and salmon in a large bowl.

2. Divide salad evenly between 4 bowls and drizzle each with 1 tablespoon of Avocado Cream Sauce.

PER SERVING Calories: 270 | Fat: 8g | Protein: 19g | Sodium: 269mg | Fiber: 6g | Carbohydrates: 34g | Sugar: 25g

Avocado Tuna Salad

You don't need bowls to serve this salad—after you scoop the avocado out of the shell you can use the peel as your serving dish!

INGREDIENTS | SERVES 4

2 medium avocados

10 ounces canned wild tuna, drained

1 celery stalk, thinly sliced

2 tablespoons chopped green onion

Juice of 1 large lemon

¼ teaspoon sea salt

¼ teaspoon black pepper

How to Choose a Ripe Avocado

An avocado is ripe when it gives slightly when you gently squeeze it.

1. Cut avocados in half lengthwise and remove pit. Scoop avocado flesh into a large bowl and save peels.

2. Add tuna, celery, and green onion to the bowl with the avocado. Mash to combine. Squeeze lemon juice over mixture and sprinkle with salt and pepper. Stir to combine.

3. Scoop an even amount of the tuna mixture into avocado peels and serve.

PER SERVING Calories: 303 | Fat: 20.5g | Protein: 23g | Sodium: 411mg | Fiber: 7g | Carbohydrates: 9g | Sugar: 1g

Basic Vinaigrette

Consider this basic vinaigrette recipe a blank canvas. Add fresh or dried herbs or experiment with different mustards or vinegars to come up with your own signature recipe.

INGREDIENTS | YIELDS 1 CUP; SERVING SIZE: 2 TABLESPOONS

¼ cup balsamic vinegar
1 tablespoon Dijon mustard
¼ teaspoon sea salt
¼ teaspoon black pepper
¾ cup extra virgin olive oil

When to Use Olive Oil

Olive oil is a healthy fat and it does have its place in Paleo cooking, but there are certain times when a saturated fat such as coconut oil or ghee may be better. Olive oil, because it contains high amounts of monounsaturated fats, is less stable under high heat than saturated fats. When you are lightly sautéing vegetables or making salad dressing, however, olive oil is a great choice.

1. In a medium bowl, combine all ingredients except olive oil using a whisk, blender, or immersion blender.

2. Slowly pour in olive oil while continuing to whisk or blend until oil is emulsified. Store in an airtight container in the refrigerator for up to 2 weeks. Shake well or whisk before serving.

PER SERVING Calories: 187 | Fat: 20g | Protein: 0g | Sodium: 98mg | Fiber: 0g | Carbohydrates: 1.5g | Sugar: 1g

Honey Mustard Dressing

Honey mustard dressing is more than just a salad topping. Use it as a marinade for baked chicken or as a dipping sauce for sweet potato fries.

INGREDIENTS | YIELDS 1 CUP; SERVING SIZE: 2 TABLESPOONS

½ cup Dijon mustard
2 tablespoons honey
3 tablespoons apple cider vinegar
¼ teaspoon black pepper
½ cup olive oil

1. In a medium bowl, combine all ingredients except olive oil using a whisk, blender, or immersion blender.

2. Slowly pour in olive oil while continuing to whisk or blend until oil is emulsified. Store in an airtight container in the refrigerator for up to 2 weeks. Shake well or whisk before serving.

PER SERVING Calories: 147 | Fat: 14g | Protein: 1g | Sodium: 178mg | Fiber: 0.5g | Carbohydrates: 5g | Sugar: 4.5g

Paleo Ranch Dressing

This ranch dressing builds off of the basic Paleo Mayonnaise recipe, but uses coconut milk, instead of dairy milk, to add creaminess.

INGREDIENTS | YIELDS 1 CUP; SERVING SIZE: 2 TABLESPOONS

½ cup Paleo Mayonnaise (see Chapter 8)
½ cup coconut milk
1 teaspoon garlic powder
1 teaspoon dried dill
⅛ teaspoon sea salt
⅛ teaspoon black pepper

In a medium bowl, whisk all ingredients together until well combined. Store in the refrigerator in an airtight container for up to 2 weeks.

PER SERVING Calories: 96 | Fat: 10g | Protein: 1g | Sodium: 47mg | Fiber: 0g | Carbohydrates: 1g | Sugar: 0g

Asparagus and Grape Tomato Salad Toss

Blanched asparagus spears and grape tomatoes add bright color to this delicious toss. It's a feast for your eyes and your taste buds.

INGREDIENTS | SERVES 2

4 cups asparagus spears, white tips removed and cut into 1" strips

2 cups grape tomatoes, halved

2 tablespoons balsamic vinegar

1 tablespoon extra-virgin olive oil

1. In a pot of boiling water over medium heat, blanch the asparagus spears for less than 1 minute, until bright green and still crisp. Remove from heat and shock with cold water to stop the cooking process.

2. Remove the asparagus from the pot and place in a mixing bowl.

3. Add the halved grape tomatoes to the mixing bowl, and drizzle the balsamic and olive oil over the salad.

4. Toss to coat evenly, and serve in two salad bowls.

PER SERVING Calories: 154 | Fat: 7g | Protein: 7g | Sodium: 17mg | Fiber: 8g | Carbohydrates: 19g | Sugar: 11g

Fruit Salad with Ginger and Lemon Juice

Traditional fruit salad includes a couple of fruits and melons thrown together, tossed, and served. In this version, these delicious fruits get tossed in a tasty dressing of freshly squeezed lemon juice and minced ginger.

INGREDIENTS | SERVES 2

1 large grapefruit, inside pieces removed

1 cup pineapple chunks

1 cup green seedless grapes, sliced

1 Granny Smith apple, cored, sliced, and chopped

1 cup cubed cantaloupe

1 cup cubed honeydew melon

3 tablespoons freshly squeezed lemon juice

2 tablespoons freshly grated ginger

1. In a large mixing bowl, combine all ingredients.

2. Toss to coat and combine thoroughly, and share between two salad bowls.

PER SERVING Calories: 127 | Fat: 0.55g | Protein: 2g | Sodium: 18mg | Fiber: 3g | Carbohydrates: 32g | Sugar: 25g

Citrus to Brighten Fruit Flavors

Most fruit salads are delicious just as they are, and it's pretty difficult to create a bad-tasting combination of sweet fruits. Heightening and brightening the flavors, though, is easily done with just a simple addition of citrus juice. Even if you don't particularly like lemon juice or lime juice on its own, you may find that it is the perfect addition to your fruit salads because of its amazing ability to brighten the colors and the flavors of the fruit.

Grilled Tomato and Pesto Salad

A fresh tomato salad is always tasty—but in this version you take things up a notch by grilling some of the ingredients. Give it a try as an appetizer at your next barbecue!

INGREDIENTS | SERVES 2

2 large beefsteak tomatoes, sliced in ¼" slices

1 cup prepared Paleo Pesto (see Chapter 8)

2 cups chopped romaine lettuce

1. Preheat a grill to medium heat, then spray or brush with oil.

2. Paint the tomato slices on just one side with the pesto.

3. Set the pesto-painted side of the tomatoes face-down on the grill, then paint the other side with the pesto also.

4. Grill each side for about 2–3 minutes, and remove from heat.

5. In two salad bowls, with 1 cup of the chopped romaine in each, evenly divide the grilled tomatoes, and serve.

PER SERVING Calories: 396 | Fat: 34g | Protein: 10g | Sodium: 685mg | Fiber: 3g | Carbohydrates: 13g | Sugar: 5g

Avocado Cream Sauce

This versatile avocado sauce can be served over salad, burgers, or even eggs. Add a punch of heat by throwing in a diced jalapeño pepper.

INGREDIENTS | YIELDS 1 CUP; SERVING SIZE: 2 TABLESPOONS

1 large avocado, pitted
Juice of ½ medium lime
¼ cup coconut milk
2 tablespoons water
¼ cup chopped fresh cilantro leaves
¼ teaspoon sea salt
¼ teaspoon black pepper

Combine all ingredients in a food processor with the chopping blade attached (or use an immersion blender). Process until smooth and creamy.

PER SERVING Calories: 55 | Fat: 5g | Protein: 0.5g | Sodium: 77mg | Fiber: 1.5g | Carbohydrates: 2.5g | Sugar: 0g

Simple Spinach Salad

Baby spinach leaves are so tasty on their own, they really need little else to be the perfect salad. Adding cool cucumber and crisp sunflower seeds in a light coating of extra-virgin olive oil and balsamic vinegar brings out the best in this dish.

INGREDIENTS | SERVES 2

1 tablespoon balsamic vinegar
1 tablespoon extra-virgin olive oil
2 cups baby spinach leaves, washed
1 medium cucumber, peeled and sliced
2 tablespoons toasted, unsalted sunflower seeds

1. In a large mixing bowl, whisk together the balsamic vinegar and olive oil.

2. Add the spinach leaves to the mixing bowl, and toss to coat.

3. Split the spinach salad between two bowls, and top with cucumbers and sunflower seeds.

PER SERVING Calories: 149 | Fat: 12g | Protein: 4g | Sodium: 30mg | Fiber: 2g | Carbohydrates: 10g | Sugar: 4g

CHAPTER 14

Comfort Foods

Creamy Mashed Cauliflower

Cauliflower is fun to cook with because it really picks up the flavors you add to it. By adding buttery ghee and chives to this creamy dish, you'll never know you aren't eating mashed potatoes.

INGREDIENTS | SERVES 4

1 large head cauliflower, cut into florets

2 tablespoons coconut milk

2 tablespoons vegetable stock

1 tablespoon ghee

¼ teaspoon sea salt

½ teaspoon black pepper

1 tablespoon chopped fresh chives

What If You Don't Have a Steamer Basket?

If you don't have a steamer basket, simply boil the cauliflower in a large pot of water over high heat until soft, about 10 minutes.

1. Heat 2 cups of water in a large pot over high heat. Once water is boiling, place steamer insert into pot and place cauliflower florets in steamer. Cover and steam for 10–12 minutes, until soft and tender.

2. Drain and place cauliflower into a food processor with the chopping blade attached (or return to pot if using an immersion blender).

3. Add coconut milk, vegetable stock, ghee, salt, and pepper to pot or food processor with cauliflower and process until smooth. Top with fresh chives.

PER SERVING Calories: 79 | Fat: 5g | Protein: 3g | Sodium: 209mg | Fiber: 3g | Carbohydrates: 7.5g | Sugar: 3g

Mom's Meatloaf

Meatloaf is a classic dish that was a staple in many households growing up. By omitting the bread crumbs and making your own sugar-free tomato topping, this Paleo version isn't much different than the original.

INGREDIENTS | SERVES 8

1 tablespoon melted ghee
2 pounds ground beef
1 large egg, whisked
2 tablespoons plus ½ cup tomato paste, divided
½ medium yellow onion, diced
1½ teaspoons garlic powder, divided
½ teaspoon paprika
½ teaspoon sea salt, divided
1 teaspoon black pepper, divided
½ cup water
2 tablespoons apple cider vinegar
½ teaspoon allspice

1. Heat oven to 375°F. Grease a loaf pan with ghee and set aside.

2. In a large bowl, combine ground beef, egg, 2 tablespoons tomato paste, onion, 1 teaspoon garlic powder, paprika, ¼ teaspoon salt, and ½ teaspoon pepper. Use your hands to mix everything together until well combined.

3. Spread mixture evenly into prepared pan. Bake for 50 minutes. Remove from oven and drain any excess liquid from pan.

4. While meatloaf is baking, combine remaining tomato paste, water, apple cider vinegar, allspice, and remaining garlic powder, salt, and pepper in a small saucepan over medium-low heat. Simmer for 10 minutes, stirring often.

5. Spread sauce over the top of the cooked meatloaf. Return to oven and cook for an additional 10 minutes.

PER SERVING Calories: 244 | Fat: 13.5g | Protein: 24g | Sodium: 393mg | Fiber: 1g | Carbohydrates: 5g | Sugar: 3g

Classic Pot Roast

Pot roast takes time to cook properly, but it is worth the wait. Save this dish for an evening when you have time to relax while it cooks.

2 tablespoons ghee
3 pounds beef chuck pot roast
1 teaspoon garlic powder
1 teaspoon dried oregano
¼ teaspoon sea salt
¼ teaspoon black pepper
1 medium white onion, chopped
2 cloves garlic, minced
1 cup beef stock
4 large carrots, chopped
4 large parsnips, chopped
1 long sprig fresh rosemary

Varying Your Protein

During pregnancy, it is important to consume protein from a variety of sources, such as poultry, seafood, eggs, and red meat, because they all provide different nutrients. For example, fish is higher in omega-3 fatty acids and red meat is rich in vitamin B_{12}.

1. Preheat oven to 325°F. Heat ghee in a large oven-safe pot or Dutch oven over medium-high heat.

2. Season chuck roast on all sides with garlic powder, oregano, salt, and pepper. Add chuck roast to pot and sear for 2–3 minutes per side, until all sides are browned. Remove from pot and set aside.

3. Add onion and garlic to pot and cook, stirring often, for 3–4 minutes, until onion begins to soften. Add stock, carrots, and parsnips to pot. Stir to combine and bring to a boil.

4. Once boiling, remove from heat; place roast in the center of the pot on top of vegetables and top with rosemary sprig. Cover and cook in the oven, undisturbed, for 2½ hours, until meat and vegetables are tender.

5. Remove rosemary sprig. Slice or shred roast and serve with vegetables.

PER SERVING Calories: 439 | Fat: 27g | Protein: 35g | Sodium: 248mg | Fiber: 3g | Carbohydrates: 12g | Sugar: 4g

Smoky Sweet Potato Soup

This puréed soup is overflowing with flavor and gets its creaminess from coconut milk.

INGREDIENTS | SERVES 8

4 cups vegetable stock

2 medium sweet potatoes, peeled and cut into large cubes

1 cup fresh or canned pumpkin purée

½ medium yellow onion, diced

2 garlic cloves, minced

1 chipotle pepper in adobo sauce, diced, plus 1 tablespoon of adobo sauce

1 cup coconut milk

½ cup water

1 tablespoon cinnamon

1 teaspoon nutmeg

¼ teaspoon sea salt

¼ teaspoon black pepper

1. In a large saucepan over medium-high heat, add vegetable stock, sweet potatoes, pumpkin, onion, garlic, chipotle pepper, and adobo sauce. Allow mixture to come to a boil and then reduce heat to medium-low and simmer for about 20 minutes, until potatoes are fork tender.

2. Transfer soup to a blender or use an immersion blender to blend until smooth. Return soup to saucepan over medium-low heat. Stir in coconut milk, water, cinnamon, nutmeg, salt, and pepper until warm and well combined.

3. If desired, sprinkle with additional cinnamon or chipotle powder.

PER SERVING Calories: 110 | Fat: 6g | Protein: 2g | Sodium: 385mg | Fiber: 2.5g | Carbohydrates: 13.5g | Sugar: 4g

Paleo Stuffin' Muffins

You won't find traditional stuffing on a Paleo holiday table, but these mini handheld stuffing muffins make a perfect stand-in.

INGREDIENTS | SERVES 4

1 tablespoon melted coconut oil

½ pound ground Italian sausage

½ pound ground beef

½ medium yellow onion, diced

2 celery stalks, diced

1 carrot, diced

4 button mushrooms, diced

1 large egg, beaten

½ cup almond meal

1 tablespoon dried sage

1 teaspoon dried thyme

1 teaspoon garlic powder

⅛ teaspoon sea salt

¼ teaspoon black pepper

Even More Holiday Flavor

If you are serving these around the holidays, stir in ½ cup of dried cherries or cranberries before transferring to muffin tins.

1. Preheat oven to 350°F. Grease a muffin tin with the coconut oil or use a silicone muffin pan.

2. Add remaining ingredients to a large bowl. Using your hands, mix until everything is well incorporated.

3. Scoop about ⅓ cup of the mixture into each muffin tin. Bake for 30–35 minutes, until meat is cooked through and muffins are golden brown on top.

PER SERVING Calories: 420 | Fat: 32g | Protein: 25g | Sodium: 515mg | Fiber: 3g | Carbohydrates: 8g | Sugar: 3g

Cinnamon Baked Sweet Potato

Slow roasting sweet potatoes makes them even sweeter in this couldn't-be-simpler recipe.

INGREDIENTS | SERVES 4

2 medium sweet potatoes
1 tablespoon coconut oil
1 teaspoon cinnamon
¼ teaspoon sea salt

Don't Throw Out That Skin!

When you eat a baked sweet potato in the skin, you are getting more fiber, vitamins, and minerals than when you eat only the flesh.

1. Preheat oven to 425°F. Scrub and rinse potatoes and dry well. Poke potatoes 5 or 6 times with a fork and place on a large foil-lined baking sheet.

2. Bake for 45–60 minutes, until tender. Potatoes are done when they can easily be pierced with a knife and they are soft throughout.

3. Slice potatoes in half lengthwise. Drizzle with coconut oil and sprinkle with cinnamon and sea salt.

PER SERVING Calories: 87 | Fat: 3g | Protein: 1g | Sodium: 183mg | Fiber: 2g | Carbohydrates: 13.5g | Sugar: 3g

Spaghetti Squash Marinara

You may be surprised by how much spaghetti squash resembles traditional spaghetti noodles, but the real surprise is how much healthier this dish is!

INGREDIENTS | SERVES 4

1 large spaghetti squash
½ cup water
1 pound ground beef
2 cups pasta sauce (check label for added sweeteners and preservatives)
¼ teaspoon sea salt
¼ teaspoon black pepper

How Do You Like Your Spaghetti?

Top this Paleo spaghetti dish as you would traditional spaghetti. Try sliced black olives, red pepper flakes, or chopped fresh basil leaves.

1. Preheat oven to 375°F. Cut spaghetti squash in half lengthwise and use a spoon to scoop out the seeds. Place squash, cut side down, in a large glass baking dish. Pour water into dish and bake until tender, 40–45 minutes.

2. When squash is cool enough to handle, use a fork to scrape the flesh away from the skin and place strands in a large serving bowl. Set aside.

3. While squash is cooking, heat a large skillet over medium heat. Add ground beef and cook until completely browned, 8–10 minutes. Stir often with a spoon or spatula to break meat up as it cooks.

4. When meat is cooked through, turn heat to medium-low and stir in pasta sauce, salt, and pepper. Cook, stirring occasionally, until sauce is heated through, 3–4 minutes. Pour meat and sauce mixture into serving bowl over spaghetti squash.

PER SERVING Calories: 342 | Fat: 15g | Protein: 27g | Sodium: 738mg | Fiber: 6g | Carbohydrates: 25g | Sugar: 16g

Pizza-Stuffed Bell Peppers

Craving pizza? You can give in to your craving and stick to your Paleo diet with these sausage-stuffed peppers. They contain many of the same toppings as a typical supreme pizza.

INGREDIENTS | SERVES 4

4 large bell peppers, any color
2 tablespoons coconut oil
½ medium red onion, diced
2 cloves garlic, minced
1 pound ground Italian sausage
4 button mushrooms, diced
10 kalamata olives, sliced
½ cup tomato sauce
¼ cup tomato paste
1 teaspoon crushed red pepper
1 teaspoon chopped fresh thyme
1 teaspoon chopped fresh oregano
⅛ teaspoon sea salt
⅛ teaspoon black pepper

A Good Source of Lycopene

Studies have shown that lycopene, the cancer-fighting carotenoid that gives tomatoes their red hue, is actually better absorbed by the body from cooked tomato products such as tomato sauce or paste than from raw tomatoes.

1. Heat oven to 400°F.

2. Cut tops off peppers; dice the tops and remove seeds from the peppers.

3. Heat coconut oil in a large pan over medium heat. Add onions to pan and cook until translucent, stirring often, 2–3 minutes. Add garlic and cook for 1 minute, while continuing to stir. Add sausage, diced pepper tops, and mushrooms to pan. Cook until sausage is browned, 8–10 minutes, stirring occasionally to break up meat.

4. Drain meat mixture and add to a large bowl along with olives, tomato sauce, tomato paste, crushed red pepper, thyme, oregano, salt, and black pepper. Stir well to combine.

5. Scoop an even amount of filling into each bell pepper. Stand peppers up in a small glass baking dish and bake for 40–45 minutes, until peppers are tender and filling is heated through.

PER SERVING Calories: 482 | Fat: 37g | Protein: 20g | Sodium: 1,080mg | Fiber: 4.5g | Carbohydrates: 19g | Sugar: 8g

CHAPTER 15

Smoothies

Pumpkin Pie Smoothie

Like pumpkin pie in a glass, this smoothie makes a great quick breakfast or post-workout treat!

INGREDIENTS | SERVES 2

1 (15-ounce) can pumpkin purée

1 medium banana, sliced and frozen

4 ice cubes

1 cup coconut milk

1 cup water

½ teaspoon cinnamon

1 teaspoon pumpkin pie spice

Add all ingredients to a blender and blend until smooth. Divide evenly between 2 large glasses.

PER SERVING Calories: 348 | Fat: 25g | Protein: 5g | Sodium: 29mg | Fiber: 8g | Carbohydrates: 34g | Sugar: 14g

A Healthy Treat!

The cinnamon in this smoothie gives it a real nutritional boost. Cinnamon helps to regulate blood sugar, keeping your energy levels steady and even all day long.

Mint Chocolate Smoothie

This smoothie tastes like a chocolatey mint dessert and it even has a slight green hue thanks to the avocado.

INGREDIENTS | SERVES 2

1 medium avocado, peeled and pitted

4 ice cubes

1 cup coconut milk

1 cup water

2 tablespoons unsweetened cocoa powder

¼ teaspoon peppermint extract

¼ teaspoon vanilla extract

Add all ingredients to a blender and blend until smooth. Divide evenly between 2 large glasses.

PER SERVING Calories: 397 | Fat: 40g | Protein: 5g | Sodium: 23mg | Fiber: 8.5g | Carbohydrates: 15g | Sugar: 1g

Banana Berry Smoothie

This smoothie is a great way to use up frozen fruit you may have in your freezer. Use a bag of mixed berries or any berries you have on hand.

INGREDIENTS | SERVES 2

1 medium banana, sliced and frozen

1½ cups frozen mixed berries

1 tablespoon molasses

1 cup coconut milk

1 cup water

1 teaspoon cinnamon

Add all ingredients to a blender and blend until smooth. Divide evenly between 2 large glasses.

PER SERVING Calories: 372 | Fat: 25g | Protein: 4g | Sodium: 20mg | Fiber: 5g | Carbohydrates: 41.5g | Sugar: 24g

A Healthy Alternative to Table Sugar

Molasses retains all of the minerals that are lost when sugar cane is refined to make white sugar. Among other minerals, molasses is high in iron, copper, calcium, and magnesium.

Tropical Mango Smoothie

This smoothie provides a taste of the tropics—perfect for a hot summer day.

INGREDIENTS | SERVES 2

1 cup frozen pineapple chunks

1½ cups frozen mango chunks

1 medium orange, peeled and quartered

4 ice cubes

1 cup coconut milk

1 cup water

1 teaspoon powdered ginger

Add all ingredients to a blender and blend until smooth. Divide evenly between 2 large glasses.

PER SERVING Calories: 378 | Fat: 25g | Protein: 4g | Sodium: 18mg | Fiber: 5g | Carbohydrates: 43g | Sugar: 33g

Hidden Greens Banana Smoothie

The spinach in this smoothie may make it look green, but it tastes just like cinnamon-sweet banana.

INGREDIENTS | SERVES 2

2 medium bananas, sliced and frozen
½ cup coconut milk
¾ cup water
2 large handfuls spinach
4 ice cubes
1 teaspoon cinnamon

Add all ingredients to blender and blend until smooth. Divide evenly between 2 large glasses.

PER SERVING Calories: 226 | Fat: 12.5g | Protein: 3g | Sodium: 32mg | Fiber: 4g | Carbohydrates: 30.5g | Sugar: 14.5g

Cherry Chocolate Smoothie

High in antioxidants, cocoa is a not-so-sinful treat. Studies also show that cocoa may lower blood pressure and cholesterol.

INGREDIENTS | SERVES 2

1 medium banana, sliced and frozen
1½ cups frozen cherries
4 ice cubes
2 tablespoons unsweetened cocoa powder
1 cup coconut milk
1 cup water

Add all ingredients to blender and blend until smooth. Divide evenly between 2 large glasses.

PER SERVING Calories: 341 | Fat: 25.5g | Protein: 5g | Sodium: 17.5mg | Fiber: 5g | Carbohydrates: 32.5g | Sugar: 18g

Cucumber Citrus Green Smoothie

This refreshing smoothie combines the natural powers of grapefruit, spinach, and cucumbers for a mix of immunity-boosting vitamins and minerals. It's great as an afternoon snack or a pick-me-up when you're feeling fatigued.

INGREDIENTS | SERVES 2

1 cup chopped spinach

2 medium cucumbers, peeled

1 medium grapefruit, peeled and deseeded

1 cup ice (optional)

1. Combine spinach, cucumbers, and grapefruit in a blender.

2. Blend thoroughly and add ice until desired consistency is achieved.

PER SERVING Calories: 69 | Fat: 1g | Protein: 2g | Sodium: 16mg | Fiber: 3g | Carbohydrates: 15g | Sugar: 12g

Mango Blend Smoothie

Sweet and bursting with vitamins from mangos, pineapples, and romaine, this green drink provides healthy doses of fiber to keep you full and focused throughout the day.

INGREDIENTS | SERVES 2

1 cup chopped romaine lettuce

1 cup mango chunks, peeled and deseeded

1 cup pineapple chunks

1 cup coconut milk

1 cup ice

Combine all ingredients in a blender and blend until desired consistency is reached.

PER SERVING Calories: 140 | Fat: 3g | Protein: 1g | Sodium: 2mg | Fiber: 3g | Carbohydrates: 28g | Sugar: 24g

Energy-Booster Smoothie

Carrots, spinach, and apples combine for a delightfully sweet, filling, and energy-boosting smoothie. They provide important vitamins and minerals needed to keep you healthy and to nurture your growing baby.

INGREDIENTS | SERVES 3

1 cup chopped spinach
4 medium carrots, peeled, and chopped
2 medium apples, peeled and cored
2 cups water

1. Place spinach, carrots, apples, and 1 cup of water in a blender and blend until thoroughly combined.

2. Add remaining 1 cup of water, as needed, while blending until desired consistency is achieved.

PER SERVING Calories: 87 | Fat: 0g | Protein: 1g | Sodium: 64mg | Fiber: 4g | Carbohydrates: 22g | Sugar: 15g

Apple Pie Smoothie

Smooth, satisfying, and aromatic, this smoothie packs all the healthiest ingredients into a tasty treat that will calm your craving for apple pie! This a great guilt-free treat to share with friends, too.

INGREDIENTS | SERVES 2

3 medium apples, cored

1 medium banana, peeled

1 teaspoon cinnamon

1 teaspoon cloves

1 teaspoon nutmeg

1 teaspoon ginger

1 teaspoon vanilla

2 cups coconut milk

2 cups ice

1. Slice apples and layer in a shallow baking dish. Add enough water to cover the bottom of the baking dish, and bake at 375°F for 20–30 minutes or until apples are fork tender.

2. Combine cooked apples, banana, cinnamon, cloves, nutmeg, ginger, vanilla, and coconut milk in the blender with ½ cup of the ice and blend until thoroughly combined.

3. Add remaining ice gradually while blending until desired consistency is reached.

PER SERVING Calories: 279 | Fat: 9g | Protein: 3.8g | Sodium: 407mg | Fiber: 8g | Carbohydrates: 52g | Sugar: 32g

CHAPTER 16

Desserts

No-Bake Brownie Bites

These rich, chocolatey brownie bites are quite addictive, so share them with a loved one and watch them disappear.

INGREDIENTS | YIELDS 24 BITES; SERVING SIZE: 2 BITES

14 Medjool dates, pitted

1 teaspoon vanilla extract

4 tablespoons unsweetened cocoa powder

½ cup shelled pistachios

½ cup pecans

½ cup unsweetened, shredded coconut (optional)

Ingredient Comparison

These little brownie bites have only six ingredients. Next time you are at the grocery store, flip over a box of packaged brownies and see if you can count the ingredients. You'll probably tire of counting before you reach the end of the list.

1. Add dates, vanilla, and cocoa powder to a food processor with the chopping blade attached. Process on high until the mixture forms a paste. Add nuts to food processor and process until finely chopped and well incorporated with date mixture (you may need to break the mixture up with a fork if it starts to form a ball).

2. Using your hands, roll the dough into 1" balls. Spread the shredded coconut onto a large plate. Roll each of the balls into the coconut until evenly coated. Serve immediately or refrigerate until ready to serve.

PER SERVING Calories: 104 | Fat: 7g | Protein: 2g | Sodium: 1mg | Fiber: 2.5g | Carbohydrates: 11g | Sugar: 7g

Cocoa Mint Cookies

With these minty cookies, you can start a healthful holiday family baking tradition.

INGREDIENTS | YIELDS 18 COOKIES; SERVING SIZE: 2 COOKIES

1 cup almond flour
1 tablespoon coconut flour
¼ cup cocoa powder
⅛ teaspoon sea salt
½ teaspoon baking soda
1 teaspoon peppermint extract
½ teaspoon vanilla extract
¼ cup melted coconut oil
2 tablespoons maple syrup

1. Preheat oven to 350°F. Line a baking sheet with parchment paper.

2. In a large bowl, stir together almond flour, coconut flour, cocoa powder, sea salt, and baking soda.

3. In a medium bowl, whisk together peppermint extract, vanilla extract, coconut oil, and maple syrup. Pour wet ingredients into bowl with dry ingredients and whisk until smooth.

4. Scoop dough by rounded tablespoons and place on a large baking sheet about 2" apart (use two baking sheets if necessary). Bake for 10–12 minutes. Allow to cool for 5 minutes on baking sheet, then transfer to a wire cooling rack to cool completely.

PER SERVING Calories: 144 | Fat: 12.5g | Protein: 3g | Sodium: 104mg | Fiber: 2.5g | Carbohydrates: 7.5g | Sugar: 3g

Loaded Paleo Brownies

When you bite into these dense, fudgy brownies, your taste buds will be treated to a special surprise thanks to the dried cherries and chopped pecans.

INGREDIENTS | YIELDS 9 BROWNIES

3 tablespoons melted coconut oil, divided

⅓ cup unsweetened cocoa powder

½ teaspoon baking soda

¼ teaspoon sea salt

1 cup almond butter

⅓ cup maple syrup

1 large egg, whisked

1 teaspoon vanilla extract

¼ cup unsweetened dried cherries

¼ cup chopped pecans

Brownies à la Mode

If you have a craving for brownies and ice cream, serve these brownies with a scoop of Quick Banana Soft Serve (see recipe in this chapter). Allow brownies to cool completely before topping with soft serve so it doesn't melt too quickly.

1. Preheat oven to 325°F. Grease a 9" × 9" glass baking dish with 1 tablespoon of coconut oil.

2. In a large bowl, stir together cocoa powder, baking soda, and sea salt.

3. In a separate large bowl, whisk together almond butter, maple syrup, egg, remaining 2 tablespoons coconut oil, and vanilla extract.

4. Pour wet ingredients into bowl with dry ingredients and whisk until smooth. Using a spatula, fold in cherries and pecans.

5. Pour brownie batter into prepared baking dish and bake for 20–25 minutes, until a toothpick inserted into the center comes out clean. Allow to cool completely before cutting.

PER SERVING Calories: 280 | Fat: 22g | Protein: 9g | Sodium: 276mg | Fiber: 3g | Carbohydrates: 16.5g | Sugar: 10.5g

Quick Banana Soft Serve

You don't need an ice cream maker to make this cool treat. Slice and freeze your bananas early in the day so they'll be ready when you are.

INGREDIENTS | SERVES 4

4 medium bananas, sliced and frozen
1 teaspoon vanilla extract
½ teaspoon cinnamon
2 teaspoons coconut milk

1. Remove banana slices from freezer and allow them to thaw for 5–10 minutes.

2. Add bananas, vanilla, and cinnamon to a food processor with the chopping blade attached. Turn on food processor and slowly pour in coconut milk through ingredient spout. Continue to process until mixture is smooth and resembles soft serve ice cream.

PER SERVING Calories: 113 | Fat: 1g | Protein: 1g | Sodium: 1mg | Fiber: 3g | Carbohydrates: 27g | Sugar: 14.5g

Individual Peach and Apricot Cobbler

Dessert for one! If a sweet craving hits but you don't want to make a full pan of cookies or brownies, try this fruity, grain-free cobbler!

INGREDIENTS | SERVES 1

1 medium peach, pitted and diced
6 unsulfured dried apricots
1 teaspoon melted coconut oil
1 teaspoon cinnamon, divided
¼ teaspoon nutmeg
¼ teaspoon ground cloves
1 teaspoon vanilla, divided
2 tablespoons almond meal
1 tablespoon shredded coconut
1 tablespoon finely chopped walnuts
1 tablespoon ghee, softened to room temperature
1 tablespoon honey

Almond Meal versus Almond Flour

Is there really a difference between almond meal and almond flour? Technically speaking, no. The terms can be used interchangeably. However, you will usually find almond flour to be made from blanched almonds, and it has a finer consistency. Try sifting almond meal before using it for baking if the consistency seems uneven.

1. Preheat oven to 350°F.

2. In a small ramekin, combine peach, apricots, coconut oil, ½ teaspoon cinnamon, nutmeg, ground cloves, and ½ teaspoon vanilla. Stir well to incorporate spices and coat peaches with coconut oil. Place ramekin on a baking sheet and bake for 5 minutes.

3. While filling is baking, mix together almond meal, shredded coconut, chopped walnuts, and remaining cinnamon in a small bowl. Add remaining vanilla and ghee. Using your hands or a fork, mix ghee around until well combined with other topping ingredients and a crumble forms.

4. Remove ramekin from oven. Drizzle peaches with honey and spread evenly with crumb topping. Return to oven for an additional 12–15 minutes, until crumb topping is just beginning to brown.

PER SERVING Calories: 544 | Fat: 32g | Protein: 7g | Sodium: 8mg | Fiber: 9g | Carbohydrates: 65g | Sugar: 54g

Coco-nutty Frozen Blueberries

This chilled treat is reminiscent of the chocolate bark often seen around the holidays, but with the flavors of coconut and fresh berries.

INGREDIENTS | SERVES 8

1 cup coconut butter

1 tablespoon coconut oil

1 teaspoon honey (optional)

1 teaspoon cinnamon

½ cup frozen blueberries

2 tablespoons unsweetened shredded coconut

What Is Coconut Butter?

Coconut butter is puréed coconut flesh with a consistency similar to smooth almond butter. Like coconut oil, it can be more solid or more liquid depending on the room temperature. You can make coconut butter at home or buy it in many grocery stores or online.

1. In a small saucepan over medium-low heat, combine coconut butter, coconut oil, honey, and cinnamon. Cook, stirring often, until it reaches a creamy consistency, 3–4 minutes.

2. Evenly spread coconut butter into a parchment paper–lined 8" × 8" square pan. Press frozen blueberries into mixture and sprinkle with shredded coconut. Place in the refrigerator to cool for 15–20 minutes, until coconut butter hardens. Break apart into bite-sized pieces and serve immediately or store in the refrigerator.

PER SERVING Calories: 214 | Fat: 18g | Protein: 8g | Sodium: 148mg | Fiber: 2.5g | Carbohydrates: 8g | Sugar: 4g

Fruity Avocado Ice Pops

A cool, summery treat that is actually good for you! If you don't have Popsicle-sized molds, you can use ice cube trays and make bite-sized pops.

INGREDIENTS | YIELDS 6 POPS

2 medium avocados, pitted
½ cup coconut milk
½ cup freshly squeezed orange juice
2 tablespoons honey
1 teaspoon powdered ginger

1. Place all ingredients in a food processor with the chopping blade attached and process until smooth.

2. Pour mixture into 6 ice pop molds and freeze until solid, about 2 hours.

PER SERVING Calories: 177 | Fat: 14g | Protein: 2g | Sodium: 8mg | Fiber: 4.5g | Carbohydrates: 14.5g | Sugar: 8g

Sautéed Cinnamon Bananas

Sautéing these cinnamon-coated bananas in coconut oil enhances their natural sweetness.

INGREDIENTS | SERVES 2

2 large bananas, cut into ½" thick slices
1 teaspoon cinnamon
2 tablespoons coconut oil

1. Sprinkle banana slices on both sides with cinnamon.

2. Heat coconut oil in a medium pan over medium-high heat. Once pan is hot, add banana slices in an even layer in the pan and sauté for 1–2 minutes per side, until soft and golden.

PER SERVING Calories: 244 | Fat: 14g | Protein: 1.5g | Sodium: 1mg | Fiber: 4g | Carbohydrates: 32g | Sugar: 16.5g

Slow-Cooked Pineapple

Slow cooking makes pineapple meltingly tender—perfect for dessert any night of the week.

INGREDIENTS | SERVES 8

1 whole pineapple, peeled

1 vanilla bean, split

3 tablespoons water

Place all ingredients into a large slow cooker. Cook on low for 4 hours or until fork tender. Remove the vanilla bean before serving.

PER SERVING Calories: 57 | Fat: 0g | Protein: 1g | Sodium: 1mg | Fiber: 2g | Carbohydrates: 15g | Sugar: 11g

Pumpkin Pie Pudding

This is a flavorful, festive, and favorite holiday treat. Serve warm, or use as a fun dip for sliced fruit.

INGREDIENTS | SERVES 8

1 (15-ounce) can pumpkin purée, softened

1 (12-ounce) can coconut milk

¾ cup honey

½ cup almond meal

2 large eggs, beaten

2 tablespoons coconut butter, melted

2 tablespoons honey

2 teaspoons pumpkin pie spice

1 teaspoon coconut extract

1. In a large bowl stir together pumpkin and ¼ cup of the coconut milk, stirring until well blended with the pumpkin.

2. Add remaining coconut milk and the remaining ingredients, and beat until blended.

3. Transfer to a 3–4-quart slow cooker, coated with non-stick cooking spray.

4. Cover and cook on low for 6–8 hours, until pudding is set when lightly touched with finger.

PER SERVING Calories: 271 | Fat: 14g | Protein: 5g | Sodium: 27mg | Fiber: 2g | Carbohydrates: 38g | Sugar: 33g

Orange Pudding Cake

Creamsicle and Orange Julius fans will love this dessert. It also works well with lemon juice and lemon zest instead of the orange. The beaten egg whites act as the leavening; the pudding forms on the bottom as the cake cooks.

INGREDIENTS | SERVES 6

4 large eggs, separated
⅓ cup fresh orange juice
1 tablespoon orange zest, grated
3 tablespoons coconut butter, softened
1½ cups coconut milk
1 cup almond flour
1 cup honey

1. Add the egg yolks, orange juice, orange zest, and coconut butter to a food processor; process for 30 seconds to cream the ingredients together. Continue to process while you slowly pour in the coconut milk.

2. In a medium bowl, combine the almond flour and honey. Stir to mix.

3. Pour the egg yolk mixture into the bowl and stir to combine it.

4. Add the egg whites to a separate chilled bowl; whip until stiff peaks form. Fold into the cake batter.

5. Pour into a greased small slow cooker. Cover and cook on low for 2–2½ hours or until the cake is set on top.

PER SERVING Calories: 445 | Fat: 25g | Protein: 10g | Sodium: 57mg | Fiber: 2g | Carbohydrates: 54g | Sugar: 49g

CHAPTER 17

Snacks

Paleo Trail Mix Bars

Sweet and chewy with a little crunch, these bars have the texture of traditional granola bars. They also make a perfect snack for you when you are feeding your new baby!

INGREDIENTS | YIELDS 12 BARS

2 large eggs, beaten

1 teaspoon vanilla

1 tablespoon honey

½ cup shredded unsweetened coconut

½ cup raw sunflower seeds

1 cup chopped almonds

1 cup chopped walnuts

½ cup raisins

2 tablespoons sea salt

1 teaspoon cinnamon

Little Seed, Big Nutrition

Sunflower seeds are small, but mighty! They are a good source of protein, healthy fats, vitamin E, magnesium, and selenium.

1. Preheat oven to 350°F. Line a 9" × 9" glass baking dish with parchment paper.

2. In a small bowl, stir together eggs, vanilla, and honey until well combined.

3. In a large bowl, stir together shredded coconut, sunflower seeds, almonds, walnuts, raisins, salt, and cinnamon.

4. Pour egg mixture into bowl with dry ingredients and stir until everything is evenly coated. Pour into prepared dish and press down evenly until tightly packed.

5. Bake for 18–20 minutes. Let cool completely and cut into 12 bars.

PER SERVING Calories: 193 | Fat: 15g | Protein: 6g | Sodium: 1,192mg | Fiber: 3g | Carbohydrates: 11g | Sugar: 6g

Plantain Chips

Need a chip for your salsa and guacamole? Look no further than these oven-roasted plantain chips.

INGREDIENTS | SERVES 4

2 large green plantains
1 tablespoon melted coconut oil
½ teaspoon sea salt

Benefits of Oven-Roasting

Oven-roasting chips requires much less oil than deep-frying. You still get the fatty-acid benefits, but with far fewer calories.

1. Preheat oven to 350°F. Line a large baking sheet with parchment paper and set aside.

2. Cut the tips off of the plantains and discard. Make a slit all the way along the length of the peel, being careful not to cut through the actual plantain, and carefully pull peel away.

3. Slice plantains as thinly as possible and toss in a large bowl with coconut oil and sea salt.

4. Spread in an even layer on prepared baking sheet and bake for 20–25 minutes, until golden and crispy. Serve within 1 or 2 days to preserve freshness.

PER SERVING Calories: 139 | Fat: 4g | Protein: 1g | Sodium: 298mg | Fiber: 2g | Carbohydrates: 28.5g | Sugar: 13g

Crispy Kale Chips

Feel free to add your own flavors to these munchable chips. You could try garlic powder, chili pepper, or even cinnamon and nutmeg—whatever your taste buds are craving!

INGREDIENTS | SERVES 4

1 large bunch dinosaur, or Tuscan, kale (about 1 pound), stems removed and coarsely chopped
1 tablespoon melted ghee
⅛ teaspoon sea salt
¼ teaspoon black pepper

1. Preheat oven to 450°F.

2. In a large bowl, toss kale with ghee, salt, and pepper. Arrange kale in an even layer on a wire cooling rack set over a baking sheet.

3. Roast until kale just begins to crisp, 10–12 minutes.

PER SERVING Calories: 84 | Fat: 4g | Protein: 3.5g | Sodium: 122mg | Fiber: 2g | Carbohydrates: 11g | Sugar: 0g

Fruity Trail Mix

Skip the junk at the convenience store and bring along this tasty road-trip snack.

INGREDIENTS | SERVES 12

1 cup raw almonds
½ cup raw cashews
½ cup unsweetened dried cherries
½ cup dried pineapple chunks
¼ cup raw pumpkin seeds
1 teaspoon cinnamon
⅛ teaspoon sea salt

Add all ingredients to a large freezer bag or storage container. Shake well to combine.

PER SERVING Calories: 95 | Fat: 7g | Protein: 3.5g | Sodium: 25mg | Fiber: 1.5g | Carbohydrates: 5.5g | Sugar: 2g

Snack Attack

This recipe makes a large batch of trail mix. If you don't feel like sharing, portion it out into snack-sized bags or storage containers and keep a little with you everywhere you go so you'll be ready when hunger hits.

Grain-Free Carrot Cake Muffins

You'll never miss the cream cheese frosting when you bite into these soft and chewy carrot cake muffins.

INGREDIENTS | YIELDS 12 MUFFINS

4 tablespoons melted ghee, divided
2¼ cups almond flour
½ teaspoon baking soda
¼ teaspoon sea salt
2 teaspoons ground cinnamon
1 teaspoon ground nutmeg
½ teaspoon allspice
½ teaspoon ground cloves
½ teaspoon ground ginger
3 large eggs, beaten
2 tablespoons honey
1 tablespoon vanilla extract
1 medium carrot, grated
½ cup raisins
½ cup chopped walnuts
¼ cup unsweetened shredded coconut

1. Preheat oven to 350°F. Grease a muffin pan with 1 tablespoon melted ghee or use a silicone muffin pan.

2. In a large bowl, stir together almond flour, baking soda, salt, cinnamon, nutmeg, allspice, cloves, and ginger.

3. In a separate large bowl, whisk together remaining ghee, eggs, honey, and vanilla until smooth.

4. Pour wet ingredients into bowl with dry ingredients and whisk until smooth. Fold in carrot, raisins, walnuts, and coconut.

5. Pour ¼ cup of batter into each muffin tin so they are about ¾ full. Bake muffins for 18–20 minutes, until a toothpick inserted into the center comes out clean.

PER SERVING Calories: 240 | Fat: 20g | Protein: 7g | Sodium: 125mg | Fiber: 3.5g | Carbohydrates: 11.5g | Sugar: 5g

Berry Mojito Salad

This pregnancy-friendly mojito-flavored fruit salad is alcohol free, but contains all the flavor of the popular Cuban drink.

INGREDIENTS | SERVES 8

Juice of 1 medium lime plus 1 tablespoon lime zest

Small handful fresh mint leaves, very thinly sliced

⅛ teaspoon sea salt

1 cup blackberries

1 cup blueberries

1 cup quartered strawberries

1 cup raspberries

1 cup watermelon cubes

1. In a small bowl combine lime zest, mint leaves, and sea salt and set aside.

2. In a large bowl combine blackberries, blueberries, strawberries, raspberries, and watermelon.

3. Squeeze lime juice over fruit and sprinkle with lime zest mixture. Toss until well mixed.

PER SERVING Calories: 40 | Fat: 0g | Protein: 1g | Sodium: 41mg | Fiber: 3g | Carbohydrates: 9.5g | Sugar: 5.5g

The Easiest Way to Slice Herbs

Thinly slicing mint (or other herb) leaves doesn't have to be tricky. The technical term is "chiffonade" and it is easy to do. Stack the leaves on top of each other, roll tightly, and cut the rolled leaves into thin slices.

Coco-Bananas with Cashew Butter

This filling treat is packed with protein, making it a perfect pre- or post-workout snack!

INGREDIENTS | SERVES 1

1 medium banana

1½ tablespoons cashew butter

2 tablespoons cold coconut milk

¼ teaspoon cinnamon

Slice banana into a small bowl. Spoon cashew butter on top, drizzle with coconut milk, and sprinkle with cinnamon.

PER SERVING Calories: 304 | Fat: 18.5g | Protein: 8g | Sodium: 115mg | Fiber: 5g | Carbohydrates: 33g | Sugar: 16.5g

Paleo BLT

Bacon, lettuce, and tomato are all perfectly Paleo. Wrap it all up and you've got yourself one tasty "sandwich."

INGREDIENTS | SERVES 2

4 slices bacon

4 large romaine lettuce leaves

1 medium tomato, chopped

2 tablespoons Paleo Mayonnaise (see Chapter 8)

1. Add bacon to a large cold skillet and heat over medium heat. Cook until evenly browned and beginning to crisp, flipping often, about 7–10 minutes. Remove to a paper towel–lined plate to drain.

2. Top each romaine lettuce leaf with 1 slice of bacon, some chopped tomato, and ½ tablespoon of Paleo Mayonnaise. Wrap and serve!

PER SERVING Calories: 375 | Fat: 36g | Protein: 8g | Sodium: 390mg | Fiber: 2g | Carbohydrates: 5g | Sugar: 2g

Sweet and Spicy Walnuts

These nuts are a perfect sweet and savory snack, guaranteed to please just about any palate.

INGREDIENTS | SERVES 12

2 tablespoons coconut oil

¼ cup honey

1 teaspoon ground ginger

1 teaspoon curry powder

½ teaspoon cayenne

¼ teaspoon onion powder

¼ teaspoon garlic powder

3 cups shelled walnuts

1. Pour coconut oil into a small slow cooker, turn on high, and allow to melt.

2. While oil is melting, in a separate bowl mix honey and seasonings together.

3. Once oil has melted, add walnuts to slow cooker and stir. Add honey and seasoning blend to slow cooker, and stir until evenly coated.

4. Cover and cook on high for 1 hour. Stir the nuts, re-cover, and cook for another hour.

5. Remove cover and cook an additional 20–30 minutes, until the nuts are dry. Cool and store in airtight containers.

PER SERVING Calories: 214 | Fat: 19g | Protein: 5g | Sodium: 1mg | Fiber: 2g | Carbohydrates: 10g | Sugar: 7g

CHAPTER 18

Soups, Stews, and Stocks

Kitchen Sink Soup

This recipe gets its name because you really can use any vegetables you have lying around and it is hard to go wrong . . . throw in everything but the kitchen sink!

INGREDIENTS | SERVES 8

6 cups Basic Chicken Stock (see recipe in this chapter)

4 large boneless, skinless chicken breasts (about 2 pounds)

1 large yellow onion, chopped

1 small head cauliflower, cut into florets

1 large zucchini, sliced

1 large red bell pepper, chopped

2 large carrots, sliced

2 ribs celery, sliced

1 (14.5-ounce) can fire-roasted diced tomatoes, drained

2 tablespoons chopped fresh parsley

1 teaspoon fresh thyme leaves

2 garlic cloves, minced

¼ teaspoon sea salt

½ teaspoon black pepper

Add all ingredients to a large slow cooker and cook on low for 6–8 hours, until chicken is cooked through. Shred chicken with a fork before serving.

PER SERVING Calories: 240 | Fat: 5.5g | Protein: 31g | Sodium: 573mg | Fiber: 3g | Carbohydrates: 16.5g | Sugar: 8g

What If You Don't Have a Slow Cooker?

If you don't have a slow cooker, instead you can precook and shred your chicken. Sauté onions and garlic in 2 tablespoons of ghee in a large stockpot. Then pour in the remaining vegetables and shredded chicken and sprinkle with herbs and spices. Bring to a boil, reduce heat to medium-low, and simmer for 20 minutes until vegetables are soft.

Basic Chicken Stock

Keep a container of this versatile chicken stock in your refrigerator or freezer at all times, as it can be used as a base for many Paleo recipes.

INGREDIENTS | YIELDS 12 CUPS; SERVING SIZE: 1 CUP

1 chicken carcass (left over from a roasted chicken) or 2 pounds of chicken pieces (bone-in and skin-on)

1 large white onion, quartered

2 carrots, chopped

2 ribs celery, chopped

2 garlic cloves, smashed

2 bay leaves

2 sprigs fresh thyme

2 sprigs fresh rosemary

12 cups water

1. Place chicken carcass in a large slow cooker and arrange vegetables around chicken. Scatter herbs around vegetables and cover with water. Cook on low for 8–10 hours.

2. Turn off heat and strain using a fine sieve or cheese-cloth so you are left with only the liquid. Store in the refrigerator for 2–3 days or in the freezer for up to 3 months.

PER SERVING Calories: 86 | Fat: 3g | Protein: 6g | Sodium: 320mg | Fiber: 0g | Carbohydrates: 5g | Sugar: 2g

Finding High-Quality Chicken at a Great Price

Many butchers or local farms will sell chicken pieces, such as necks and backs, for very low prices because they are usually the pieces nobody wants—but they are perfect for making chicken stock!

Basic Vegetable Stock

This is a flavorful broth that is low in sodium and high in disease-fighting phytochemicals. Try adding mushrooms for additional flavor.

**INGREDIENTS | YIELDS 1 GALLON;
SERVING SIZE: 1 CUP**

2 pounds yellow onions

1 pound carrots

1 pound celery

1 bunch fresh parsley stems

1½ gallons water

4 stems fresh thyme

2 bay leaves (fresh or dried)

10–20 peppercorns

Homemade Stocks

Your homemade stocks give a special quality to all the dishes you add them to. Not only will the flavor of homemade stocks be better than that from purchased bases, but you will have added your own personal touch to the meal. Always cook them uncovered, as covering will cause them to become cloudy.

1. Peel and roughly chop the onions and carrots. Roughly chop the celery (stalks only; no leaves) and fresh parsley stems.

2. Put the vegetables and water in a stockpot over medium heat; bring to a simmer and cook, uncovered, for 1½ hours.

3. Add the herbs and peppercorns, and continue to simmer, uncovered, for 45 minutes. Adjust seasonings to taste as necessary.

4. Remove from heat and cool by submerging the pot in a bath of ice and water. Strain using a fine sieve or cheesecloth so you are left with only the liquid. Place in freezer-safe containers and store in the freezer until ready to use.

PER SERVING Calories: 15 | Fat: 0g | Protein: 0g | Sodium: 0mg | Fiber: 0g | Carbohydrates: 3g | Sugar: 2g

Beef Stock

Try lining the strainer with cheesecloth before pouring the soup through. In addition to straining out all the solids, this is helpful in removing any extra fat from the stock.

INGREDIENTS | YIELDS 1 GALLON; SERVING SIZE: 1 CUP

5–6 pounds beef with bones
1 tablespoon ghee
5 medium yellow onions, chopped
2 shallots, chopped
1 pound carrots, chopped
1 bunch celery, chopped
1½ gallons water
5 sprigs fresh thyme or 1 tablespoon dried
½ bunch fresh parsley or 1 tablespoon dried
3 bay leaves

1. Remove the beef from the bones. Rinse the beef and pat dry with paper towels.

2. Heat the ghee in a large stockpot over medium heat. Add the beef and brown the meat on all sides. Add the onions, shallots, carrots, and celery and sauté for 2 minutes.

3. Add the water, thyme, parsley, and bay leaves. Bring to a simmer and cook for 8 hours, uncovered.

4. Strain the broth through a fine-meshed sieve, and discard the solids. Use immediately, or let cool completely and freeze for later use.

PER SERVING Calories: 38 | Fat: 1g | Protein: 5g | Sodium: 70mg | Fiber: 0g | Carbohydrates: 3g | Sugar: 1g

Fish Stock

Do not use oily fish bones such as those from salmon or tuna. Light whitefish bones are a better option for this stock.

INGREDIENTS | YIELDS 1 GALLON; SERVING SIZE: 1 CUP

4 pounds fish bones
3 large yellow onions, chopped
2 large carrots, chopped
3 stalks celery, chopped
½ bunch fresh parsley
8 sprigs fresh thyme
3 bay leaves
¼ teaspoon freshly cracked black pepper
2 gallons cold water

1. Rinse the fish bones in ice-cold water.

2. Place all the ingredients in a large stockpot and bring to a simmer. Cook over medium-low heat for 2 hours, uncovered.

3. Strain the broth through a fine-meshed sieve, and discard the solids. Use in recipe as needed, or let cool completely and store for later use.

PER SERVING Calories: 20 | Fat: 1g | Protein: 1g | Sodium: 85mg | Fiber: 0g | Carbohydrates: 3g | Sugar: 2g

Taco Soup

Slow cooker soups make dinnertime a breeze, and the leftovers can be frozen for later use. Top with diced avocado for a serving of healthy fat.

INGREDIENTS | SERVES 8

1 red onion, chopped

2 pounds ground beef

1 cup salsa verde

5 cups Basic Vegetable Stock (see recipe in this chapter)

4 garlic cloves, minced

2 (4-ounce) cans fire-roasted green chiles

2 (14.5-ounce) cans diced fire-roasted tomatoes

¼ teaspoon garlic powder

¼ teaspoon onion powder

¼ teaspoon red pepper flakes

¼ teaspoon dried oregano

½ teaspoon paprika

1 teaspoon ground cumin

¼ teaspoon sea salt

¼ teaspoon black pepper

Add all ingredients to a large slow cooker. Cook on low for 6–8 hours. Stir to break up meat before serving.

PER SERVING Calories: 252 | Fat: 11.5g | Protein: 25g | Sodium: 834mg | Fiber: 2g | Carbohydrates: 13g | Sugar: 7g

Should You Brown Meat Before Adding It to the Slow Cooker?

Browning meat does enhance its flavor, but it isn't necessary. If you aren't in a hurry, you can brown the meat and onions in a sauté pan with 2 tablespoons of cooking fat before adding to slow cooker with other ingredients.

Moroccan Lamb Stew

The exotic flavors in this stew make it taste much more complicated to make than it actually is. The leftovers will taste even better the next day when the seasonings have had more time to mingle.

INGREDIENTS | SERVES 8

1 teaspoon cumin

1 teaspoon dried ginger

½ teaspoon cinnamon

¼ teaspoon turmeric

¼ teaspoon saffron threads

¼ teaspoon sea salt

½ teaspoon black pepper

3 pounds lamb stew meat, cut into 1" cubes

4 tablespoons ghee

1 large yellow onion, chopped

2 cups Beef Stock (see recipe in this chapter)

4 large carrots, chopped

1 (14.5-ounce) can diced tomatoes

1 cup dried apricots, chopped

1. In a large bowl, stir together the cumin, ginger, cinnamon, turmeric, saffron, salt, and pepper. Add lamb to bowl and toss to coat.

2. Heat ghee in a large pot over medium heat. Add onion and cook until softened, stirring occasionally, about 5 minutes. Add lamb to pot and cook, stirring every 2–3 minutes, until all sides are browned.

3. Pour in beef stock and stir in carrots, tomatoes, and apricots. Bring to a boil and reduce heat to medium-low. Simmer for 30 minutes, until meat is cooked through and vegetables are soft.

PER SERVING Calories: 360 | Fat: 16g | Protein: 37g | Sodium: 400mg | Fiber: 3g | Carbohydrates: 18g | Sugar: 12.5g

Sour Cherry Beef Stew

This recipe was adapted from a traditional beef stew recipe. You will be surprised at how good this Paleo version tastes.

INGREDIENTS | SERVES 10

¼ cup almond flour

½ teaspoon nutmeg

1 teaspoon cinnamon

½ teaspoon allspice

½ teaspoon ground black pepper

2 pounds chuck steak, cubed

2 tablespoons ghee

2 medium onions, chopped

2 (16-ounce) cans sour cherries (reserve half of the juice)

2 cups Beef Stock (see recipe in this chapter)

2 pounds button mushrooms, quartered

½ cup water

1. Combine almond flour, nutmeg, cinnamon, allspice, and pepper in a plastic bag.

2. Add chuck steak to plastic bag and shake to coat evenly.

3. Heat ghee in a large skillet over medium-high heat.

4. Sear steak quickly in skillet for 1–2 minutes each side. Remove from skillet and place in slow cooker.

5. Using the same skillet, cook onion over medium heat for 8 minutes.

6. Add cherries and half the cherry juice to the skillet and cook for 5 more minutes, until the onions are browned. Pour cherry mixture into slow cooker.

7. Add stock, mushrooms, and water to a large slow cooker. Cook for at least 5 hours on low heat in slow cooker. Stir in the remaining cherry juice before serving.

PER SERVING Calories: 295 | Fat: 13g | Protein: 22g | Sodium: 203mg | Fiber: 4g | Carbohydrates: 25g | Sugar: 17g

Creamy Butternut Squash Soup

This dish combines the warm, delicious flavors of the fall harvest into a creamy blended soup.

INGREDIENTS | SERVES 8

1 large butternut squash, peeled, chopped, and seeded

2 tablespoons melted coconut oil, divided

¼ teaspoon sea salt, divided

1 teaspoon black pepper, divided

1 large yellow onion, chopped

2 Granny Smith apples, peeled and chopped

5 cups Basic Vegetable Stock (see recipe in this chapter)

1 teaspoon chopped fresh sage leaves

1 teaspoon cinnamon

¼ teaspoon nutmeg

1 cup coconut milk

Take a Shortcut

In a hurry or can't find butternut squash at your grocery store or farmers' market? Most grocery stores carry butternut squash cubes in the frozen vegetable section.

1. Preheat oven to 400°F. In a large bowl, toss butternut squash with 1 tablespoon coconut oil, ⅛ teaspoon salt, and ¼ teaspoon pepper. Place on a baking pan and roast for 25 minutes, until soft, stirring once after 10 minutes.

2. Heat remaining tablespoon of coconut oil in a large soup pot over medium heat. Add onion to pot and cook, stirring occasionally, until softened, about 3 minutes. Add the roasted squash, apples, stock, sage, cinnamon, nutmeg, and remaining salt and pepper. Stir well to combine.

3. Turn heat to medium-high and allow soup to come to a boil. Reduce heat to medium-low and simmer until squash and apples are tender, 30–40 minutes. Purée with an immersion blender (or transfer to a blender and blend until smooth). Pour in coconut milk and blend again until combined.

PER SERVING Calories: 145 | Fat: 9.5g | Protein: 1.5g | Sodium: 424mg | Fiber: 2g | Carbohydrates: 16g | Sugar: 7g

Sage and Squash Soup

Sweet squash combines with aromatic and tasty sage in this soup, a healthy way to satisfy any cravings. In addition, this homemade delight is completely devoid of poor ingredients that most canned varieties would include.

INGREDIENTS | SERVES 4

4 cups water

3 cups cubed summer squash, peeled, seeds removed

2 teaspoons sea salt

½ cup dried sage leaves

Brighten Flavors with Spices

There are certain ingredients that are well known for being brighteners of tastes and flavors. Spices such as sage fall into this category. Summer squash is a delicious vegetable with a light, buttery, nutty taste that improves dramatically when seasoned. (Many herbs are actually more powerful in their dried versions, so rather than opting for fresh in soups, opt for dried spices, unless the spice is a garnish.)

1. Bring the water to a boil in a large pot over medium heat.

2. Reduce heat to low, add the squash, salt, and sage, and simmer for about 20–25 minutes, or until fork tender.

3. Using an immersion blender, emulsify the squash and sage until no bits remain.

4. Serve hot or cold, and garnish with crushed walnuts or crumbled sage leaves.

PER SERVING Calories: 26 | Fat: 0.66g | Protein: 2g | Sodium: 1,188mg | Fiber: 2.5g | Carbohydrates: 5g | Sugar: 2g

Summer-Style Vegetarian Chili

This light, meat-free chili is full of an array of summer vegetables, high in fiber, and loaded with vitamins and minerals.

INGREDIENTS | SERVES 8

1 bulb fennel, diced

4 radishes, diced

2 stalks celery, diced, including leaves

2 large carrots, cut into coin-sized pieces

1 medium onion, diced

1 shallot, diced

4 cloves garlic, sliced

1 habanero pepper, diced

12 ounces tomato paste

½ teaspoon dried oregano

½ teaspoon black pepper

½ teaspoon crushed rosemary

½ teaspoon cayenne

½ teaspoon ground chipotle

1 teaspoon chili powder

1 teaspoon tarragon

¼ teaspoon cumin

¼ teaspoon celery seed

2 medium zucchini, cubed

2 medium summer squash, cubed

10 Campari tomatoes, quartered

1. In a large slow cooker add the fennel, radishes, celery, carrots, onion, shallot, garlic, habanero, tomato paste, and all the spices. Stir.

2. Cook on low for 6–7 hours; then stir in the zucchini, summer squash, and tomatoes. Cook on high for an additional 30 minutes. Stir before serving.

PER SERVING Calories: 109 | Fat: 1g | Protein: 5g | Sodium: 386mg | Fiber: 7g | Carbohydrates: 24g | Sugar: 13g

Pork and Apple Stew

If you prefer a tart apple taste, you can substitute Granny Smith apples for the Golden Delicious. (You can also add more apples if you wish. Apples and pork were made for each other!)

INGREDIENTS | SERVES 8

1 (3-pound) boneless pork shoulder roast

⅛ teaspoon freshly ground black pepper, or to taste

1 large sweet onion, diced

2 Golden Delicious apples, peeled, cored, and diced

1 (2-pound) bag baby carrots

2 stalks celery, finely diced

2 cups apple juice (fresh or 100% juice, no sugar added)

2 tablespoons honey (optional)

½ teaspoon dried thyme

¼ teaspoon ground allspice

¼ teaspoon dried sage

2 large sweet potatoes, peeled and quartered

1. Trim the roast of any fat; discard the fat and cut the roast into bite-sized pieces. Add the roast to a large slow cooker along with the remaining ingredients in the order given. (You want to rest the sweet potato quarters on top of the mixture in the slow cooker.)

2. Cover and cook on low for 6 hours or until the roast is cooked through and tender.

PER SERVING Calories: 326 | Fat: 12g | Protein: 34g | Sodium: 226mg | Fiber: 4g | Carbohydrates: 18g | Sugar: 12g

Herbs and Spice Test

If you're unsure about the herbs and spices suggested in a recipe, wait to add them until the end of the cooking time. Once the meat is cooked through, spoon out ¼ cup or so of the pan juices into a microwave-safe bowl. Add a pinch of each herb and spice (in proportion to how they're suggested in the recipe), microwave on high for 15–30 seconds, and then taste the broth to see if you like it. Season the dish accordingly.

CHAPTER 19

Fresh Juices

Apple Watermelon Punch

This simple juice is hydrating and delicious—and will calm any sweet cravings you may experience in a healthy, natural way.

2 large apples, cored

3 cups watermelon, cut into chunks

How Much Produce Should I Buy to Juice?

When juicing, follow this rule when you're planning your shopping list: 1 pound of produce will yield approximately 1 cup of juice.

1. Process the apples through an electronic juicer according to the manufacturer's directions.

2. Add the watermelon.

3. Whisk the juice together to combine and serve immediately.

PER SERVING Calories: 242 | Fat: 1g | Protein: 3.4g | Sodium: 4.5mg | Carbohydrates: 62g | Sugar: 50g

Nectarine Cooler

This refreshing juice is packed with beta carotene, an antioxidant that can protect your body from free radical damage. In addition, your body converts beta carotene into vitamin A, which helps build and maintain healthy bones, skin, teeth, and soft tissue.

INGREDIENTS | YIELDS 1 CUP

4 nectarines, pitted

1 medium carrot, trimmed

1 orange, peeled

Choosing Oranges for Juicing

Some oranges are bred for ease of eating, like the easy peeling navel. But other oranges yield more juice. Valencia is a great choice; Hamlins and blood oranges also yield more juice per fruit.

1. Process the nectarines through your electronic juicer according to the manufacturer's directions.

2. Add the carrot, followed by the orange segments.

3. Stir or shake the juice thoroughly to combine the ingredients and serve.

PER SERVING Calories: 318 | Fat: 1.9g | Protein: 7g | Sodium: 49mg | Carbohydrates: 76g | Sugar: 56g

Tropical Cucumber Juice

Cucumber contains silica, a trace mineral that helps provide strength to the connective tissues of the skin. Cucumbers help with water retention, and are high in vitamins A and C as well as folic acid, which is crucial for healthy brain and spine development in your baby.

INGREDIENTS | YIELDS 2 CUPS

1 cup pineapple, peeled, cored, and cut into chunks
1 medium mango, pitted
1 medium cucumber, peeled
½ lemon, rind intact

1. Process the pineapple through your electronic juicer according to the manufacturer's directions.

2. Add the mango, followed by the cucumber.

3. Cut lemon into thin slices and add it last.

4. Stir the juice well before serving.

PER SERVING Calories: 270 | Fat: 1g | Protein: 4g | Sodium: 12mg | Carbohydrates: 70g | Sugar: 52g

Apple Plum Juice

This juice is terrific for occasional constipation problems, and is rich in vitamins and phytonutrients, too.

INGREDIENTS | YIELDS 1 CUP

2 large apples, cored
4 black plums, pitted

1. Process the fruits in any order through an electronic juicer according to the manufacturer's directions.

2. Serve alone or over ice.

PER SERVING Calories: 227 | Fat: 1g | Protein: 2.4g | Sodium: 0mg | Carbohydrates: 58g | Sugar: 58g

Minty Melon Cooler

All melons are good for you because of their high water content. Cantaloupe is especially good, as it also contains high levels of beta carotene.

Alkaline Veggies Can Detox the Body

Juice from alkaline vegetables, including carrots, tomatoes, parsley, spinach, kale, and celery, helps detoxify the liver, kidneys, blood, and muscle tissue of toxins that have been accumulating for years.

1. Cut the melon into chunks and process through an electronic juicer according to the manufacturer's directions.

2. Roll the mint and parsley into balls to compress and add to the juicer.

3. Add the blueberries.

4. Whisk the juice together to combine ingredients and enjoy!

PER SERVING Calories: 193 | Fat: 1.2g | Protein: 4.6g | Sodium: 60mg | Carbohydrates: 46g | Sugar: 36g

Vegetable Super Juice

Add a generous dash of hot sauce to this juice for extra zip! It's great on the rocks as a refreshing side to a summer lunch.

INGREDIENTS | YIELDS 1½ CUPS

1 whole medium cucumber
6 leaves romaine lettuce
4 stalks of celery, including leaves
2 cups fresh spinach
½ cup alfalfa sprouts
½ cup fresh parsley

Sandy Spinach?

Spinach grows best in sandy soils, but can be tough to really rinse well. Rather than rinsing spinach through a colander, place it in a deep bowl or kettle and cover it with water. Gently toss to allow any sand or grit to fall to the bottom and lift the greens out.

1. Cut the cucumber into pieces and process through your juicer according to the manufacturer's directions.

2. Wrap the lettuce leaves around the celery stalks and add to the feeding tube.

3. Add the spinach, sprouts, and parsley in any order you desire.

4. Mix the juice thoroughly before serving.

PER SERVING Calories: 127 | Fat: 1.5g | Protein: 8g | Sodium: 212mg | Carbohydrates: 25g | Sugar: 10g

Orange Strawberry Banana Juice

Always remember that the nutrients in fresh juice are fragile. Every minute the juice stands, you lose enzymes and other micronutrients. Retain the full benefits of your freshly made juice by drinking them as soon as possible after you make them.

INGREDIENTS | YIELDS 1½ CUPS

1 large orange, peeled
1 cup strawberries
1 medium banana, peeled

1. Process the orange and the strawberries through an electronic juicer according to the manufacturer's directions.

2. Add the banana and transfer to a blender until the mixture is smooth. Serve immediately.

PER SERVING Calories: 237 | Fat: 1g | Protein: 4g | Sodium: 2mg | Carbohydrates: 59g | Sugar: 38g

Three-Grape Juice

When it comes to fruit juicing, little can compare with the mighty grape! This trio provides a nice balance of flavor, as the white and red grapes balance the more intense Concords.

INGREDIENTS | YIELDS 1½ CUPS

1 cup Concord grapes
1 cup red globe grapes
1 cup white or green seedless grapes

Great Grapes

Regarded in many cultures as "the queen of fruits," grapes are incredibly rich in phytonutrients, antioxidants, vitamins, and minerals and are a rich source of micronutrient minerals like copper, iron, and manganese.

1. Process the grapes in any order through an electronic juicer according to the manufacturer's directions.

2. Serve alone or over ice.

PER SERVING Calories: 312 | Fat: 0.7g | Protein: 3.2g | Sodium: 9mg | Carbohydrates: 81g | Sugar: 70g

Ginger Celery Cooler

The distinct Asian flavor in this juice makes it perfect for a summer snack! Add the juice of 1 red bell pepper for added sweetness and a burst of vitamins A, C, and E.

INGREDIENTS | YIELDS 1 CUP

3 stalks celery, with leaves
1 small clove of fresh garlic, peeled
1 (1") piece fresh ginger
1 medium cucumber
2 scallions, trimmed

1. Process the celery through an electronic juicer according to the manufacturer's directions.

2. Add the garlic and the ginger, followed by the cucumber and the scallions.

3. Mix the juice to combine the ingredients and serve.

PER SERVING Calories: 94 | Fat: 1g | Protein: 3.7g | Sodium: 107mg | Carbohydrates: 20g | Sugar: 8g

Golden Veggie Juice

Yellow tomatoes, yellow summer squash, and yellow wax beans combine for a beautiful color and a mild, pleasing flavor.

INGREDIENTS | YIELDS 1 CUP

4 yellow pear tomatoes

1 medium yellow summer squash

1 cup fresh yellow wax beans

Let the Sunshine In

Yellow fruits and vegetables are teeming with carotenoids and bioflavonoids, which are a class of plant pigments that function as antioxidants. Sunny-colored foods also have an abundance of vitamin C. These nutrients will help you during your pregnancy, as they support your heart and vision, and help your digestion and immune systems. Yellow fruits and veggies help maintain healthy skin and promote stronger bones and teeth.

1. Process the tomatoes through an electronic juicer according to the manufacturer's directions.

2. Add the squash, followed by the beans.

3. Stir the juice to combine the ingredients and serve alone or over ice.

PER SERVING Calories: 232 | Fat: 1g | Protein: 14g | Sodium: 59mg | Carbohydrates: 44g | Sugar: 8.5g

Blackberry Booster

Blackberries are rich in anti-inflammatory agents, which can help with joint pain or with conditions such as arthritis. They also help reduce puffy eyes and skin.

INGREDIENTS | YIELDS 1½ CUPS

2 cups blackberries
1 cup blueberries
½ cup raspberries

Blackberry Benefits

The high tannin content of blackberries helps tighten tissue, relieve intestinal inflammation, and reduce hemorrhoids and stomach disorders.

1. Process the blackberries through an electronic juicer according to the manufacturer's directions.

2. Add the blueberries and raspberries.

3. Stir or shake the juice to combine the ingredients and enjoy!

PER SERVING Calories: 240 | Fat: 2.2g | Protein: 5.8g | Sodium: 5mg | Carbohydrates: 56g | Sugar: 31g

Tangy Gazpacho Juice

Here is the pure juice form of the traditional cold soup. Most of the fiery heat of fresh jalapeños can be avoided if you carefully remove the seeds and ribs of the pepper before juicing. If it's too much for your stomach to handle, you can omit the jalapeño entirely.

INGREDIENTS | YIELDS 2 CUPS

2 large tomatoes
½ green pepper, seeded
½ red pepper, seeded
1 fresh jalapeño pepper, seeded
4 scallions, trimmed
1 clove garlic, peeled

1. Process the tomatoes through an electronic juicer according to the manufacturer's directions.

2. Add the peppers, followed by the scallions and the garlic.

3. Whisk or shake the juice to combine the ingredients and serve over ice.

PER SERVING Calories: 107 | Fat: 1.6g | Protein: 4.8g | Sodium: 28mg | Carbohydrates: 23g | Sugar: 14g

Raspberry Peach Passion

This juice is so delicious, you'll want some every day! Passion fruit is rich in fiber, potassium, and vitamins A and C.

INGREDIENTS | YIELDS 1½ CUPS

2 large peaches, pitted
1 cup raspberries
1 cup passion fruit pulp

Choosing the Best Passion Fruit

Choose fruits that are well ripened, plump, and heavy for their size. Fruits with a lightly wrinkled skin are actually more flavorful. Scoop out the pulp and discard the tough shell.

1. Process the peaches through your electronic juicer according to the manufacturer's directions.

2. Add the raspberries, followed by the passion fruit.

3. Stir or shake the juice thoroughly to combine ingredients and serve over ice.

PER SERVING Calories: 329 | Fat: 2g | Protein: 9g | Sodium: 67mg | Carbohydrates: 93g | Sugar: 51g

APPENDIX A

Nutritious Pregnancy and Postpartum Meal Plan

Pregnancy can be unpredictable. You may be craving a big, juicy burger one minute and unable to be in the same room as one the next. During pregnancy, it is essential that you are getting enough nutrients, calories, and water. Let your body be your guide. If you are still hungry, have a little more. If you are feeling nauseated, eat what you can or wait a couple of hours and see if anything sounds appetizing. This 28-day meal plan includes lots of variety to meet your ever-changing needs (and cravings and aversions). Each day consists of three meals and two snacks, but feel free to change up when you eat, based on your hunger and daily plans. For example, if you'll be eating lunch and then heading out to the gym, bring one of your snacks for a post-workout recovery meal.

Another benefit of this meal plan is that it helps you to utilize leftovers. Each recipe in the book includes the servings per recipe. Pay attention to these numbers and adjust as needed so you can have leftovers ready to go instead of always having to prepare a meal when you are busy (or just need a nap).

This meal plan is perfect for new moms, too. Your body needs a nutrient-dense diet to help you recover and to keep your energy up while caring for a newborn. Remember, too, that if you are breastfeeding you need about an extra 500 calories per day to support your milk supply.

This meal plan should serve as a guide to provide you with a variety of choices and help you shop for and prepare your meals and snacks for the week, but only you (and your health care provider) can know exactly how much and which types of food are right for you.

28-DAY MEAL PLAN

Day	Breakfast	Snack	Lunch	Snack	Dinner
Day 1	Garden Veggie Omelet with 1/2 avocado	Apple and handful of nuts	Turkey Roll-Ups with Paleo Mayonnaise	Plantain Chips, baby carrots, and salsa	Moroccan Lamb Stew
Day 2	Ginger Carrot Breakfast Casserole	Paleo Trail Mix Bar and a banana	Leftover Moroccan Lamb Stew	Crispy Kale Chips and a hard-boiled egg	Broiled Tilapia with Pistachio Cherry Sauce and sautéed zucchini
Day 3	Leftover Ginger Carrot Breakfast Casserole	Hidden Greens Banana Smoothie	Avocado Tuna Salad	Banana with 2 tablespoons almond butter	Slow Cooker Pulled Pork over roasted sweet potato with salsa verde
Day 4	Banana Pancakes with 1 tablespoon chopped walnuts and 1/2 cup fresh berries	Baby carrots and Tropical Fruit Salsa	Leftover Slow Cooker Pulled Pork with bell peppers, Plantain Chips, and Avocado Cream Sauce	Grain-Free Carrot Cake Muffin and 1/2 cup pineapple chunks	Farmers' Market Chicken Bake
Day 5	Leftover Farmers' Market Chicken Bake	Paleo Trail Mix Bar and 1 cup grapes	Salmon and Citrus Salad	Celery with Eggplant Dip (Baba Ghanoush)	Lettuce-Wrapped Bison Burger with Baked Sweet Potato Fries
Day 6	Fried Apple and Eggs with 1 chicken sausage link	Fruit Kebab and beef jerky	Leftover Lettuce-Wrapped Bison Burger with Baked Sweet Potato Fries	Banana Berry Smoothie	Garlic Rainbow Chard with Butternut Squash and Salmon.
Day 7	2 Grain-Free Carrot Cake Muffins and a banana	Spinach and Artichoke Dip with sliced peppers	2 Salmon Muffins and salad	1/2 cup blueberries and a handful of pecans	Turkey and Veggie Meatloaf with Cinnamon Skillet Carrots
Day 8	2 Salmon Muffins and 1/2 avocado	Leftover Cinnamon Skillet Carrots	Bell Pepper and Onion Hash with a fried egg	3 No-Bake Brownie Bites and a banana	Paleo Pumpkin Chili
Day 9	Scrambled Eggs and Chicken Sausage	Paleo BLT	Leftover Turkey and Veggie Meatloaf	Cherry Chocolate Smoothie	Leftover Paleo Pumpkin Chili
Day 10	Sweet Potato and Bacon Hash and 1/2 avocado	Hard-boiled egg and sliced turkey	California Salad	3 No-Bake Brownie Bites and 1/2 cup mixed berries	Lime Grilled Ahi Tuna with Pineapple Slaw

28-DAY MEAL PLAN

Day	Breakfast	Snack	Lunch	Snack	Dinner
Day 11	Pumpkin Pie Smoothie and a banana	Beef jerky with baby carrots	2 lettuce wraps with chicken, sliced peppers, and mustard	Fruity Trail Mix and an orange	Taco-less Taco Salad
Day 12	Mini Denver Omelets	Fruity Avocado Ice Pop	Leftover Taco-less Taco Salad	Olives and cherry tomatoes	Kitchen Sink Soup
Day 13	Leftover Mini Denver Omelets	Fruity Trail Mix and an apple	Paleo Cobb Salad	Fruity Avocado Ice Pop	Leftover Kitchen Sink Soup
Day 14	2 eggs with salsa and pumpkin seeds	Berry Mojito Salad	Avocado Tuna Salad	Loaded Paleo Brownie	Spaghetti Squash Marinara
Day 15	1 cup mixed berries with coconut milk and almonds	Leftover Berry Mojito Salad	Leftover Spaghetti Squash Marinara	Sweet and Spicy Walnuts	Smoky Sweet Potato Soup with Garlic-Roasted Broccoli
Day 16	Leftover Smoky Sweet Potato Soup	Loaded Paleo Brownie	Paleo Stuffin' Muffins	Tropical Mango Smoothie	Garlic Rainbow Chard with Butternut Squash and Salmon
Day 17	Zesty Italian Brunch Bake	2 Cocoa Mint Cookies	Cinnamon Baked Sweet Potato and 1 Italian sausage link	1 cup berries sprinkled with coconut	Summer Vegetable Haddock Bake
Day 18	Leftover Paleo Stuffin' Muffins	Paleo BLT	Sun-Dried Tomato Lamb Burger with side salad	1 apple and handful of mixed nuts	Lemon Pepper Shrimp Skewers and Roasted Squash
Day 19	Leftover Zesty Italian Brunch Bake	Grain-Free Carrot Cake Muffin and an orange	Asian Chicken and Broccoli Soup	Quick Banana Soft Serve	Leftover Sun-Dried Tomato Lamb Burger with side salad
Day 20	Zucchini and Spinach Breakfast	Bacon-Wrapped Dates	Jalapeño Lime Chicken Sliders and Classic Guacamole	Individual Peach and Apricot Cobbler	Slow Cooker Thanksgiving Turkey Breast and Harvest Brussels Sprouts
Day 21	Coco-Bananas with Cashew Butter	Leftover Jalapeño Lime Chicken Sliders	California Salad	Plantain Chips and Classic Guacamole	Baked Chicken and Peppers

28-DAY MEAL PLAN					
Day	**Breakfast**	**Snack**	**Lunch**	**Snack**	**Dinner**
Day 22	Mint Chocolate Smoothie and a banana	Bacon-Wrapped Dates	Leftover Baked Chicken and Peppers	Avocado drizzled with balsamic vinegar	Steak and Pepper Fajitas with Cauliflower Rice
Day 23	Pizza-Stuffed Bell Peppers	Raisins and pecans	Leftover Steak and Pepper Fajitas	Coco-nutty Frozen Blueberries	Creamy Butternut Squash Soup with Spicy Grilled Asparagus
Day 24	2 eggs scrambled with spinach and sun-dried tomatoes	Sautéed Cinnamon Bananas	Leftover Creamy Butternut Squash Soup	Veggie sticks and Honey Mustard Dressing	Curried Mahi Mahi
Day 25	Leftover Pizza-Stuffed Bell Peppers	Cinnamon Baked Sweet Potato	Stuffed Button Mushrooms	Baked apple with cinnamon and crushed pecans	Garlic Broccoli and Beef
Day 26	Leftover Stuffed Button Mushrooms and fried egg	Sliced strawberries with 2 tablespoons coconut butter	Easy Peasy Beef Roast	Sautéed pear slices	Leftover Garlic Broccoli and Beef
Day 27	Leftover Easy Peasy Beef Roast	Paleo Trail Mix Bar and an apple	Beef jerky, 1 hard-boiled egg, and veggie sticks with Paleo Mayonnaise	Crispy Kale Chips and an orange	Cedar Plank Salmon with Grilled Peaches
Day 28	Sweet and Spicy Sausage Stuffed Peppers	Crispy Kale Chips and watermelon	Salmon and Citrus Salad	Coco-Bananas with Cashew Butter	Persian Spiced Lamb with Carrot and Fennel Slaw

Paleo Pregnancy "Yes" and "No" Foods

Preparation is key in order to ensure a happy and healthy Paleo pregnancy. Keep your kitchen and pantry stocked with the following fresh, nutrient-dense foods to help you make the best choices during your pregnancy. Note that all fruits and vegetables should be thoroughly washed and meat and eggs should be fully cooked to reduce the risk of food-borne illnesses.

PALEO PREGNANCY "YES" FOODS		
Protein		Bacon (check label for additives)
		Bass
		Beef
		Bison
		Chicken
		Chuck steak
		Clams
		Cod
		Crab
		Crayfish
		Eggs
		Flank steak
		Game hen breasts
		Goat
		Ground beef
		Grouper
		Haddock
		Halibut
		Herring
		Lamb
		Liver (in moderation)
		Lobster
		London broil
		Marrow (beef, lamb, or goat)
		Mussels
		Orange roughy
		Oysters
		Pheasant
		Pork, lean

PALEO PREGNANCY "YES" FOODS—continued	
Protein	Pork chops and pork loin
	Quail
	Rabbit
	Red snapper
	Salmon, wild-caught
	Scallops
	Scrod
	Shrimp
	Tilapia
	Tongue (fully cooked)
	Trout
	Tuna, canned, unsalted
	Tuna, fresh
	Turkey breast
	Veal, lean
	Wild game (use caution, only from a trusted source)
Leafy Vegetables	Arugula
	Beet greens
	Bitterleaf
	Bok choy
	Broccoli rabe
	Brussels sprouts
	Cabbage
	Celery
	Chard
	Chicory
	Chinese cabbage
	Collard greens
	Dandelion

PALEO PREGNANCY "YES" FOODS—continued	
Leafy Vegetables	Endive
	Fiddlehead
	Kale
	Lettuce
	Radicchio
	Spinach
	Swiss chard
	Turnip
	Watercress
	Yarrow
Bulb and Stem Vegetables	Asparagus
	Celery
	Florence fennel
	Garlic
	Kohlrabi
	Leek
	Onion
Other Vegetables (includes sea vegetables and herbs of all types)	Artichoke
	Avocado
	Bell pepper
	Broccoli
	Cauliflower
	Cucumber
	Eggplant
	Squash
	Sweet pepper
	Tomatillo
	Tomato
	Zucchini

PALEO PREGNANCY "YES" FOODS—continued		
Fruits		Apples
		Apricots
		Bananas
		Blackberries
		Blueberries
		Cantaloupe
		Cherries
		Coconuts
		Cranberries
		Figs
		Grapefruit
		Grapes
		Guava
		Honeydew melon
		Kiwi
		Lemons
		Limes
		Mandarin oranges
		Mangos
		Nectarines
		Oranges
		Papaya
		Passion fruit
		Peaches
		Pears
		Persimmon
		Pineapple
		Plums
		Pomegranate

Fruits	Raspberries
	Rhubarb
	Star fruit
	Strawberries
	Tangerines
	Watermelon
	All other fruits are acceptable, as are dried fruits without sugar and preservatives
Fats, Nuts, Seeds, Oils, and Fatty Proteins	Almond butter
	Almonds
	Avocado
	Brazil nuts
	Cashew butter
	Cashews
	Chestnuts
	Coconut oil
	Flaxseed oil
	Hazelnuts/filberts
	Macadamia butter
	Macadamia nuts
	Olive oil
	Pecans
	Pine nuts
	Pistachios
	Pumpkin seeds
	Safflower oil
	Sesame seeds
	Sunflower butter
	Sunflower seeds
	Walnut oil and walnuts

PALEO PREGNANCY "NO" FOODS		
Legume Vegetables (except snow peas, sugar snap peas, and green beans)	✗	Azuki beans
	✗	Black beans
	✗	Black-eyed peas
	✗	Chickpeas (garbanzo beans)
	✗	Fava beans
	✗	Green peas
	✗	Guar
	✗	Kidney beans
	✗	Lentils
	✗	Lima beans
	✗	Mung beans
	✗	Navy beans
	✗	Peanut butter
	✗	Peanuts
	✗	Pinto beans
	✗	Red beans
	✗	Soybean and soy products
	✗	String beans
	✗	White beans
Dairy Foods	✗	All processed foods made with any dairy products
	✗	Butter
	✗	Cheese
	✗	Cream
	✗	Dairy spreads
	✗	Frozen yogurt
	✗	Ice cream
	✗	Ice milk
	✗	Milk, low-fat
	✗	Milk, powdered

PALEO PREGNANCY "NO" FOODS—continued		
Dairy Foods	X	Milk, skim
	X	Milk, whole
	X	Nonfat dairy creamer
	X	Yogurt
High-Mercury Fish	X	King mackerel
	X	Shark
	X	Swordfish
	X	Tilefish
Cereal Grains	X	Barley
	X	Corn
	X	Millet
	X	Oats
	X	Rice
	X	Rye
	X	Sorghum
	X	Wheat
	X	Wild rice
Cereal Grain–Like Seeds	X	Amaranth
	X	Buckwheat
	X	Quinoa
Other	X	Alcohol
	X	Caffeine (no more than 200 milligrams per day)
	X	Commercially prepared candy, baked goods, and other packaged snacks
	X	Fast food
	X	Refined sweeteners and artificial sweeteners
	X	Refined vegetable oils and hydrogenated oils
	X	Smoked Seafood
	X	Soda

Paleo Substitutions

cow's milk	coconut, almond, macadamia, or hazelnut milk
bacon	uncured bacon and meats
deli meat	fresh cut chicken or turkey breast, thinly sliced
salad dressing	oil and lemon or lime juice, homemade dressing
starch	spaghetti squash, butternut squash, acorn squash, sweet potatoes, plantains, cassava (yuca), jicama
soda	fruit-infused water, iced tea
salt	lemon juice, spices, fresh herbs
butter	nut oils, coconut butter
peanut butter	all other nut and seed butters
cookies and desserts	fresh fruit, homemade Paleo treats
chocolate	100% cocoa or cacao
commercially prepared meat	grass-fed, free-range meat
farm-raised fish	wild-caught fish

A Gentle Exercise Plan

Developing an Effective Exercise Plan

The fundamentals of exercise remain basically the same for everyone, pregnant or not. You should develop an effective fitness plan that includes a warm-up and a cool-down, with the activities of your choice in the middle. Once your doctor gives you the go-ahead to exercise, start exercising at a comfortable level that does not cause pain, shortness of breath, and/or excessive exhaustion. You should start slowly and increase your activity little by little, especially if you were not exercising regularly before becoming pregnant.

If you were an avid exerciser before pregnancy, you may need to make just a few simple adjustments in your program. You may find that you need to decrease your intensity level during pregnancy. The most effective plan is one that combines cardiovascular or aerobic exercise, strength, and flexibility exercises. It can be beneficial to find a variety of activities for your exercise plan because you might be more motivated to continue exercising throughout your pregnancy and beyond.

Warm Up and Cool Down

Warming up before you exercise and cooling down afterward is essential to an effective and safe program. Warming up for at least five to ten minutes revs up your body and gets your blood moving to prepare it for exercise. Cooling down for at least ten minutes gradually brings your heart rate and body temperature back to normal. You should never stop exercising abruptly without cooling down and slowing down your heart rate gradually.

Both a warm-up and cool-down should include some light aerobic activity followed by gentle stretching. Stretching can help to maintain your flexibility, and prevent muscle tightening and injury during exercise. Stretching during your cool-down can also help to prevent sore muscles the next day. Stretching can be great any time of the day when you need to release some muscle tension.

As with other aspects of exercise during pregnancy, stretching may require some modification to avoid possible injury. During pregnancy, the hormone relaxin causes your joints and ligaments to loosen, making delivery easier on the body. This makes it important to take some extra precautions when stretching. Stretching should always come after some type of warm-up exercise that increases your circulation and internal body temperature. Stretching without first warming up can lead to pulled or torn muscles and/or ligaments. The key to stretching during pregnancy is to go nice and easy and never bounce. Do not push a stretch to the point of pain or past your natural range of motion. Hold on to a chair for support if you need to while performing certain stretches. Be sure to take full breaths while you are stretching to keep blood flowing through your muscles.

Walking for Health

Walking can be a great low-impact aerobic activity during pregnancy. It is an exercise that is safe, easy to do, and inexpensive. If the weather is less than optimal, you can try a treadmill or roam around your local shopping mall. You can vary the pace, add moderate hills, and add distance when you need to. As with any exercise, you should start slow and increase your pace and distance as you feel you can. You can add a warm-up by walking slowly for the first five minutes and add a cool-down by using five minutes at the end to gradually decrease your pace.

Follow some of these tips for an effective walking program:

- Watch your posture as you walk. Stand up straight, lead with your chest, and use your abdominal muscles to support your back.
- Look ahead at the ground a few steps ahead of you and not straight down, which can strain your neck and spoil your posture.
- Get your arms moving to give your walk an extra cardiovascular kick. Move your arms from the shoulders, and don't swing them higher than your chest or across your body's midpoint.
- Take small strides. Long ones can hurt your hips and pelvic area, which are usually loosened by pregnancy hormones during pregnancy.
- Use a pace that is comfortable for your stage of pregnancy and keeps your heart rate at a safe and steady beat. Don't try to conquer steep hills that may send your heart rate soaring and put undue stress on your back.
- Invest in good athletic walking shoes that are comfortable, supportive, and fit your feet properly. If you have some swelling in your feet, you may need a larger size than usual.

- Avoid uneven terrain, such as beaches and trails, since your center of balance will shift as you become larger and you are more prone to falling. Avoid other dangerous terrain such as ice or wet pavement.
- If the weather outside is too hot and humid, opt to use an indoor treadmill, or walk at the mall.
- Find a walking partner. It can make walking more fun and can also be a safety net if something happens while you are walking.

Gentle Prenatal Yoga

Yoga can be a great exercise for flexibility, relaxation, muscle tone, posture, balance, breathing control, and developing concentration. All of these factors can help during pregnancy and again during delivery. Yoga combined with a low-impact cardiovascular exercise such as walking can round out a great exercise program. You can join a pregnancy yoga class or pick up a video specifically made for pregnant women. If you have never tried yoga before, be sure to start at the beginners' level. Yoga can be done at all different intensity levels, but while you are pregnant, you should concentrate on poses that are soothing, gentle, and fun. You want to make sure you avoid supine positions (positions on your back) and positions that have you lying on your belly after the third month or at any time before this if they begin to feel uncomfortable. As with any exercise program, consult with your doctor before you begin.

When taking a yoga class, look for an instructor who is specially trained in prenatal yoga. Some yoga moves can be tricky, so if you feel pain or discomfort, make needed adjustments. Do not hold poses for too long, and move into and out of yoga positions slowly and carefully to avoid any injury or lightheadedness. As you become larger in your third trimester, use a chair or other sturdy prop for support to avoid losing your balance. Equipment such as blocks and straps can help you to more easily move through different poses with better stability. Avoid poses that are difficult and that you may not be familiar with, as well as those that stretch the abdominal muscles too much. It is important to be extra careful because you are more prone to tearing and/or straining muscles and ligaments while pregnant.

Kegel Exercises

Kegel exercises can be very helpful once you get to the delivery room. Kegel, or pelvic-floor muscle, exercises are internal exercises that can be done to help strengthen the muscles that control your urethra, bladder, uterus, and rectum. This exercise strengthens the pelvic floor so that during delivery you are able to push more efficiently. Strengthening these muscles can also assist your body in recovering more quickly after delivery. They can help with bladder control problems that many women experience after childbirth.

Kegels are done most simply by contracting and holding the muscles that are used to stop the flow of urine. Try to do Kegels in sets of ten, and work up to three to four sets about three times each day. Start out slowly, and work your way up as these muscles become stronger. Make sure you are doing the exercises correctly. If you are not sure, ask your doctor.

Know Your Limits

Part of a safe exercise program is knowing your limits. You need to pay attention to your body's signals and stop when your body is telling you to stop. It's not good for you or your baby to exercise to the point of exhaustion, breathlessness, or overheating. Warning signs that tell you to stop exercising and/or to call your doctor include the following:

- Vaginal bleeding or amniotic fluid leakage
- Preterm labor or decreased fetal movement
- Dizziness or fainting, muscle weakness, or difficult or labored breathing prior to exertion
- Increased swelling in hands, feet, and/or ankles
- Headache, chest pain, calf pain or swelling
- Vomiting, nausea, or abdominal pain

Estimated Due Date Table

This chart lists due dates by month. Find the month and date on which your last menstrual period began, and then look below that line to see what your estimated due date is.

If your last period was . . .	1/1	1/2	1/3	1/4	1/5	1/6	1/7	1/8
Then your EDD is . . .	10/8	10/9	10/10	10/11	10/12	10/13	10/14	10/15
If your last period was . . .	1/9	1/10	1/11	1/12	1/13	1/14	1/15	1/16
Then your EDD is . . .	10/16	10/17	10/18	10/19	10/20	10/21	10/22	10/23
If your last period was . . .	1/17	1/18	1/19	1/20	1/21	1/22	1/23	1/24
Then your EDD is . . .	10/24	10/25	10/26	10/27	10/28	10/29	10/30	10/31
If your last period was . . .	1/25	1/26	1/27	1/28	1/29	1/30	1/31	
Then your EDD is . . .	11/1	11/2	11/3	11/4	11/5	11/6	11/7	
If your last period was . . .	2/1	2/2	2/3	2/4	2/5	2/6	2/7	2/8
Then your EDD is . . .	11/8	11/9	11/10	11/11	11/12	11/13	11/14	11/15
If your last period was . . .	2/9	2/10	2/11	2/12	2/13	2/14	2/15	2/16
Then your EDD is . . .	11/16	11/17	11/18	11/19	11/20	11/21	11/22	11/23
If your last period was . . .	2/17	2/18	2/19	2/20	2/21	2/22	2/23	2/24
Then your EDD is . . .	11/24	11/25	11/26	11/27	11/28	11/29	11/30	12/1
If your last period was . . .	2/25	2/26	2/27	2/28				
Then your EDD is . . .	12/2	12/3	12/4	12/5				
If your last period was . . .	3/1	3/2	3/3	3/4	3/5	3/6	3/7	3/8
Then your EDD is . . .	12/6	12/7	12/8	12/9	12/10	12/11	12/12	12/13
If your last period was . . .	3/9	3/10	3/11	3/12	3/13	3/14	3/15	3/16
Then your EDD is . . .	12/14	12/15	12/16	12/17	12/18	12/19	12/20	12/21
If your last period was . . .	3/17	3/18	3/19	3/20	3/21	3/22	3/23	3/24
Then your EDD is . . .	12/22	12/23	12/24	12/25	12/26	12/27	12/28	12/29
If your last period was . . .	3/25	3/26	3/27	3/28	3/29	3/30	3/31	
Then your EDD is . . .	12/30	12/31	1/1	1/2	1/3	1/4	1/5	

If your last period was . . .	4/1	4/2	4/3	4/4	4/5	4/6	4/7	4/8
Then your EDD is . . .	1/6	1/7	1/8	1/9	1/10	1/11	1/12	1/13
If your last period was . . .	4/9	4/10	4/11	4/12	4/13	4/14	4/15	4/16
Then your EDD is . . .	1/14	1/15	1/16	1/17	1/18	1/19	1/20	1/21
If your last period was . . .	4/17	4/18	4/19	4/20	4/21	4/22	4/23	4/24
Then your EDD is . . .	1/22	1/23	1/24	1/25	1/26	1/27	1/28	1/29
If your last period was . . .	4/25	4/26	4/27	4/28	4/29	4/30		
Then your EDD is . . .	1/30	1/31	2/1	2/2	2/3	2/4		
If your last period was . . .	5/1	5/2	5/3	5/4	5/5	5/6	5/7	5/8
Then your EDD is . . .	2/5	2/6	2/7	2/8	2/9	2/10	2/11	2/12
If your last period was . . .	5/9	5/10	5/11	5/12	5/13	5/14	5/15	5/16
Then your EDD is . . .	2/13	2/14	2/15	2/16	2/17	2/18	2/19	2/20
If your last period was . . .	5/17	5/18	5/19	5/20	5/21	5/22	5/23	5/24
Then your EDD is . . .	2/21	2/22	2/23	2/24	2/25	2/26	2/27	2/28
If your last period was . . .	5/25	5/26	5/27	5/28	5/29	5/30	5/31	
Then your EDD is . . .	3/1	3/2	3/3	3/4	3/5	3/6	3/7	
If your last period was . . .	6/1	6/2	6/3	6/4	6/5	6/6	6/7	6/8
Then your EDD is . . .	3/8	3/9	3/10	3/11	3/12	3/13	3/14	3/15
If your last period was . . .	6/9	6/10	6/11	6/12	6/13	6/14	6/15	6/16
Then your EDD is . . .	3/16	3/17	3/18	3/19	3/20	3/21	3/22	3/23
If your last period was . . .	6/17	6/18	6/19	6/20	6/21	6/22	6/23	6/24
Then your EDD is . . .	3/24	3/25	3/26	3/27	3/28	3/29	3/30	3/31
If your last period was . . .	6/25	6/26	6/27	6/28	6/29	6/30		
Then your EDD is . . .	4/1	4/2	4/3	4/4	4/5	4/6		

If your last period was . . .	7/1	7/2	7/3	7/4	7/5	7/6	7/7	7/8
Then your EDD is . . .	4/7	4/8	4/9	4/10	4/11	4/12	4/13	4/14
If your last period was . . .	7/9	7/10	7/11	7/12	7/13	7/14	7/15	7/16
Then your EDD is . . .	4/15	4/16	4/17	4/18	4/19	4/20	4/21	4/22
If your last period was . . .	7/17	7/18	7/19	7/20	7/21	7/22	7/23	7/24
Then your EDD is . . .	4/23	4/24	4/25	4/26	4/27	4/28	4/29	4/30
If your last period was . . .	7/25	7/26	7/27	7/28	7/29	7/30	7/31	
Then your EDD is . . .	5/1	5/2	5/3	5/4	5/5	5/6	5/7	
If your last period was . . .	8/1	8/2	8/3	8/4	8/5	8/6	8/7	8/8
Then your EDD is . . .	5/8	5/9	5/10	5/11	5/12	5/13	5/14	5/15
If your last period was . . .	8/9	8/10	8/11	8/12	8/13	8/14	8/15	8/16
Then your EDD is . . .	5/16	5/17	5/18	5/19	5/20	5/21	5/22	5/23
If your last period was . . .	8/17	8/18	8/19	8/20	8/21	8/22	8/23	8/24
Then your EDD is . . .	5/24	5/25	5/26	5/27	5/28	5/29	5/30	5/31
If your last period was . . .	8/25	8/26	8/27	8/28	8/29	8/30	8/31	
Then your EDD is . . .	6/1	6/2	6/3	6/4	6/5	6/6	6/7	
If your last period was . . .	9/1	9/2	9/3	9/4	9/5	9/6	9/7	9/8
Then your EDD is . . .	6/8	6/9	6/10	6/11	6/12	6/13	6/14	6/15
If your last period was . . .	9/9	9/10	9/11	9/12	9/13	9/14	9/15	9/16
Then your EDD is . . .	6/16	6/17	6/18	6/19	6/20	6/21	6/22	6/23
If your last period was . . .	9/17	9/18	9/19	9/20	9/21	9/22	9/23	9/24
Then your EDD is . . .	6/24	6/25	6/26	6/27	6/28	6/29	6/30	7/1
If your last period was . . .	9/25	9/26	9/27	9/28	9/29	9/30		
Then your EDD is . . .	7/2	7/3	7/4	7/5	7/6	7/7		

If your last period was . . .	10/1	10/2	10/3	10/4	10/5	10/6	10/7	10/8
Then your EDD is . . .	7/8	7/9	7/10	7/11	7/12	7/13	7/14	7/15
If your last period was . . .	10/9	10/10	10/11	10/12	10/13	10/14	10/15	10/16
Then your EDD is . . .	7/16	7/17	7/18	7/19	7/20	7/21	7/22	7/23
If your last period was . . .	10/17	10/18	10/19	10/20	10/21	10/22	10/23	10/24
Then your EDD is . . .	7/24	7/25	7/26	7/27	7/28	7/29	7/30	7/31
If your last period was . . .	10/25	10/26	10/27	10/28	10/29	10/30	10/31	
Then your EDD is . . .	8/1	8/2	8/3	8/4	8/5	8/6	8/7	
If your last period was . . .	11/1	11/2	11/3	11/4	11/5	11/6	11/7	11/8
Then your EDD is . . .	8/8	8/9	8/10	8/11	8/12	8/13	8/14	8/15
If your last period was . . .	11/9	11/10	11/11	11/12	11/13	11/14	11/15	11/16
Then your EDD is . . .	8/16	8/17	8/18	8/19	8/20	8/21	8/22	8/23
If your last period was . . .	11/17	11/18	11/19	11/20	11/21	11/22	11/23	11/24
Then your EDD is . . .	8/24	8/25	8/26	8/27	8/28	8/29	8/30	8/31
If your last period was . . .	11/25	11/26	11/27	11/28	11/29	11/30		
Then your EDD is . . .	9/1	9/2	9/3	9/4	9/5	9/6		
If your last period was . . .	12/1	12/2	12/3	12/4	12/5	12/6	12/7	12/8
Then your EDD is . . .	9/7	9/8	9/9	9/10	9/11	9/12	9/13	9/14
If your last period was . . .	12/9	12/10	12/11	12/12	12/13	12/14	12/15	12/16
Then your EDD is . . .	9/15	9/16	9/17	9/18	9/19	9/20	9/21	9/22
If your last period was . . .	12/17	12/18	12/19	12/20	12/21	12/22	12/23	12/24
Then your EDD is . . .	9/23	9/24	9/25	9/26	9/27	9/28	9/29	9/30
If your last period was . . .	12/25	12/26	12/27	12/28	12/29	12/30	12/31	
Then your EDD is . . .	10/1	10/2	10/3	10/4	10/5	10/6	10/7	

Standard U.S./Metric Measurement Conversions

VOLUME CONVERSIONS

U.S. Volume Measure	Metric Equivalent
⅛ teaspoon	0.5 milliliter
¼ teaspoon	1 milliliter
½ teaspoon	2 milliliters
1 teaspoon	5 milliliters
½ tablespoon	7 milliliters
1 tablespoon (3 teaspoons)	15 milliliters
2 tablespoons (1 fluid ounce)	30 milliliters
¼ cup (4 tablespoons)	60 milliliters
⅓ cup	90 milliliters
½ cup (4 fluid ounces)	125 milliliters
⅔ cup	160 milliliters
¾ cup (6 fluid ounces)	180 milliliters
1 cup (16 tablespoons)	250 milliliters
1 pint (2 cups)	500 milliliters
1 quart (4 cups)	1 liter (about)

WEIGHT CONVERSIONS

U.S. Weight Measure	Metric Equivalent
½ ounce	15 grams
1 ounce	30 grams
2 ounces	60 grams
3 ounces	85 grams
¼ pound (4 ounces)	115 grams
½ pound (8 ounces)	225 grams
¾ pound (12 ounces)	340 grams
1 pound (16 ounces)	454 grams

OVEN TEMPERATURE CONVERSIONS

Degrees Fahrenheit	Degrees Celsius
200 degrees F	95 degrees C
250 degrees F	120 degrees C
275 degrees F	135 degrees C
300 degrees F	150 degrees C
325 degrees F	160 degrees C
350 degrees F	180 degrees C
375 degrees F	190 degrees C
400 degrees F	205 degrees C
425 degrees F	220 degrees C
450 degrees F	230 degrees C

BAKING PAN SIZES

U.S.	Metric
8 × 1½ inch round baking pan	20 × 4 cm cake tin
9 × 1½ inch round baking pan	23 × 3.5 cm cake tin
11 × 7 × 1½ inch baking pan	28 × 18 × 4 cm baking tin
13 × 9 × 2 inch baking pan	30 × 20 × 5 cm baking tin
2 quart rectangular baking dish	30 × 20 × 3 cm baking tin
15 × 10 × 2 inch baking pan	30 × 25 × 2 cm baking tin (Swiss roll tin)
9 inch pie plate	22 × 4 or 23 × 4 cm pie plate
7 or 8 inch springform pan	18 or 20 cm springform or loose-bottom cake tin
9 × 5 × 3 inch loaf pan	23 × 13 × 7 cm or 2 lb narrow loaf or pâté tin
1½ quart casserole	1.5 liter casserole
2 quart casserole	2 liter casserole

Index